LOW HISTAMINE INSTANT POT COOKBOOK

Effortless Instant Pot Recipes to Manage Histamine Intolerance and Enjoy Stress-Free Cooking

Kingsley Klopp

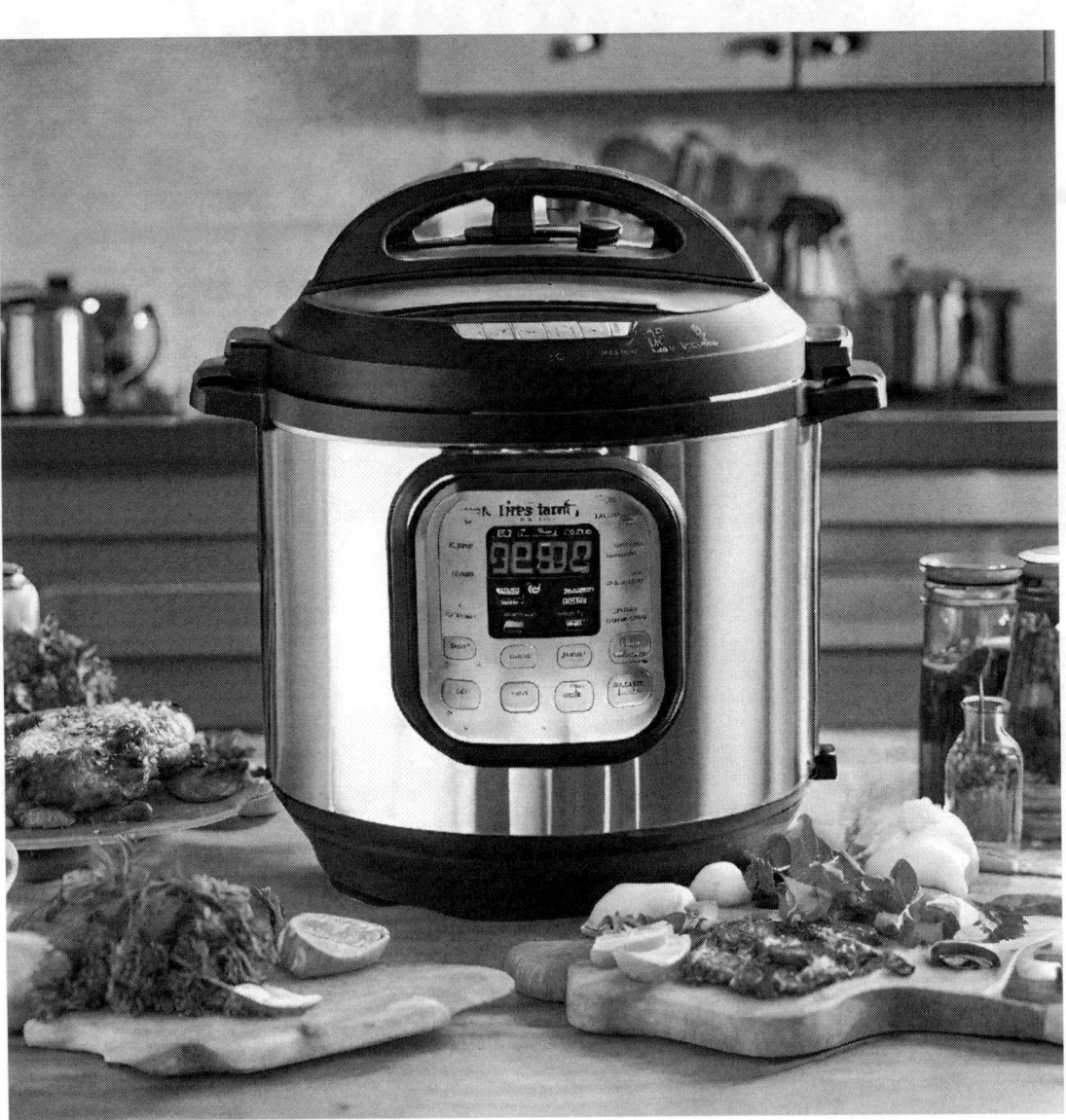

Copyright © 2024 All rights reserved.

No part of this book may be reproduced or transmitted in any form or by any means, electronic or mechanical, including photocopying, recording, or by any information storage and retrieval system, without written permission from the author. The scanning, uploading, and distribution of this book via the internet or via any other means without the permission of the author is illegal and punishable by law. The author has made every effort to ensure the accuracy of the information contained in this book. However, the author cannot be held responsible for any errors or omissions.

Table of Contents

Introduction......6

Chapter 1: Understanding Histamine
- What Is Histamine?......8
- Causes and Symptoms of Histamine Intolerance......10
- Foods High in Histamine......12
- Foods Low in Histamine......14

Chapter 2: Getting Started
- Understanding Your Instant Pot......17
- Essential Accessories......18
- Common Terms and Functions......20
- Tips for Successful Instant Pot Cooking......22
- Why Use an Instant Pot for Your Low Histamine Diet?......24

Breakfast Recipes
Quinoa Apple Cinnamon Breakfast Bowl......26
Pear and Cardamom Steel-cut Oats......27
Coconut Rice Pudding......28
Ginger-infused Millet Porridge......29
Vegetable Frittata......30
Jumbo Blueberry Pancake......31
Buckwheat Banana Pancakes......32
Savory Chicken and Rice Congee......33
Sweet Potato and Kale Hash......34
Mango Coconut Chia Pudding......35
Apple and Walnut Breakfast Quinoa......36
Pumpkin Spice Oatmeal......37
Lemon and Herb Quinoa Breakfast Pilaf......38
Instant Pot Poached Pears......39
Turkey and Sweet Potato Breakfast Casserole......40
Zucchini and Carrot Breakfast Muffins......41

Blueberry Millet Porridge..42
Spinach and Potato Breakfast Frittata.................43
Rice Flour and Coconut Pancakes.......................44
Herb-infused Breakfast Polenta............................45
Pear and Cinnamon Breakfast Bars......................46
Carrot Cake Oatmeal...47
Savory Mushroom and Rice Breakfast Bowls....48
Peachy Keen Quinoa..49

Lunch Recipes
Lemon Herb Chicken and Rice..............................50
Butternut Squash Soup..51
Beef and Sweet Potato Stew...................................52
Quinoa Stuffed Bell Peppers..................................53
Chicken and Vegetable Broth.................................54
Ginger-Lime Cauliflower Rice................................55
Parsley and Lemon Cod..56
Carrot and Cumin Soup..57
Turkey and Pumpkin Chili.....................................58
Zucchini and Basil Risotto.....................................59
Instant Pot Spaghetti Squash and Meat Sauce...60
Turkey Meatball Soup..61
Butternut Squash and Ginger Porridge................62
Sweet Potato and Chicken Curry..........................63
Lemon Garlic Shrimp and Asparagus..................64
Minty Pea Soup...65
Beef Stroganoff with Coconut Cream...................66
Herbed Chicken Salad...67
Lentil and Carrot Stew..68
Balsamic Glazed Pork Tenderloin.........................69
Instant Pot Kale and Potato Soup.........................70
Herb-Infused Turkey Breast...................................71
Quinoa Vegetable Pilaf..72
Moroccan-Inspired Chicken Stew.........................73
Beetroot and Carrot Salad......................................74
Instant Pot Lemon Pepper Cod.............................75
Saffron Rice with Vegetables..................................76

Dinner

Fennel and Orange Salad with Grilled Chicken.................77
Instant Pot Lemon Thyme Chicken................................78
Garlic-Infused Mashed Potatoes.....................................79
Bok Choy and Shiitake Mushroom Stir-Fry......................80
Basil Pesto Chicken Pasta..81
Carrot Ginger Soup..82
Turmeric Coconut Basmati Rice.....................................83
Zucchini Noodles with Olive Oil and Herbs....................84
Beef Stew with Root Vegetables....................................85
Stuffed Acorn Squash..86
Rosemary Infused Lamb Stew.......................................87
Instant Pot Fennel Chicken..88
Golden Beet Soup...89
Sage and Butter Turkey Breast.....................................90
Instant Pot Cabbage Rolls...91
Lemon-Dill Salmon Steaks..92
Root Vegetable Medley...93
Parsley-Garlic Pork Chops...94
Instant Pot Spiced Apple Cider Chicken........................95
Saffron Vegetable Couscous...96
Herbed Quinoa and Vegetable Stuffed Peppers............97
Instant Pot Maple-Glazed Chicken................................98
Instant Pot Tarragon Chicken..99
Lemon-Basil Shrimp Over Zoodles...............................100
Instant Pot Moroccan Vegetable Tagine......................101
Garlic-Infused Olive Oil Drizzled Cod..........................102

Dessert

Sticky Ginger Pudding...103
Maple Blondies..104
Vanilla Rice Pudding..105
Maple-Poached Pears..106
Coconut Custard..107
Ginger Poached Rhubarb..108
Pumpkin Spice Cake..109
Instant Pot Berry Compote..110
Peach Crumble..111

Mint and Lime Infused Mango..112
Cinnamon Applesauce...113
Blueberry Flan..114
Saffron Poached Figs..115
Pear and Ginger Jam...116
Apple and Cranberry Crisp..117
Banana Coconut Bread...118

8-WEEK MEAL PLAN..119

BONUSES..125

Dear Esteemed Reader

As you embark on the journey to rediscover the joy of cooking with our **Low Histamine Instant Pot Cookbook**, we want to share a gentle reminder about the personal nature of diet and health. Each of us is unique, and so are our dietary needs. While the recipes within these pages are crafted to help manage histamine intolerance, it's important to tailor them to suit your individual requirements. Adjust ingredients and portions as needed to fit your specific health profile and preferences.

Please consult with your healthcare provider if you're unsure about any changes or if new symptoms arise. They can offer guidance tailored to your health history and current condition, ensuring that your diet aligns perfectly with your medical needs.

Also, bear in mind that the nutritional information provided in this book is approximate. Variations in specific ingredient choices and sizes can affect the final nutritional value of each dish. We encourage you to use this information as a guide while being mindful of the potential changes depending on your ingredient selection.

Furthermore, If our cookbook has brought joy to your kitchen and table, we'd be thrilled to hear about your experiences in an Amazon review. On the flip side, if you stumble upon any hiccups while exploring our recipes, don't hesitate to get in touch at **kloppkingsley@gmail.com**. We're here to support your cooking journey every step of the way.

Introduction.

Introducing the **Low Histamine Instant Pot Cookbook**, where creativity and simplicity coexist to bring you a collection of recipes designed to make your low histamine lifestyle not only manageable but genuinely enjoyable. If you've ever felt overwhelmed by the dietary restrictions imposed by managing histamine intolerance, this cookbook is poised to become your new kitchen companion, offering a breath of fresh air and a new lease on culinary life.

Histamine intolerance can be daunting. The constant need to scrutinize labels, the struggle to balance nutrition with dietary limits, and the ever-present fear of triggering symptoms can make mealtime stressful. That's where this cookbook comes in, transforming what could be a restrictive diet into an array of appetizing and easy-to-prepare dishes. Using the beloved Instant Pot, these recipes reduce cooking time and maximize flavor, all while adhering to low histamine principles.

As to why the Instant Pot, one may wonder. This versatile kitchen gadget is a game changer for anyone, but especially for those on a specialized diet. It allows for quicker cooking times, which is essential for preserving the freshness of ingredients and minimizing histamine production that can occur in leftover foods. Whether you're simmering stews, cooking up a quick risotto, or even making dessert, the Instant Pot handles it all, locking in flavor and nutrients without the stress of constant supervision. This cookbook covers everything from the basics of what histamine intolerance is and which foods to avoid, to how to use your Instant Pot to its fullest potential. Say goodbye to lengthy prep times and hours spent over the stove. With this guide, you can whip up everything from hearty breakfasts to nourishing dinners and even indulgent desserts, all made in a way that's safe for your needs.

The recipes in this book are crafted not just with health in mind, but with an eye toward flavor and satisfaction. From the zesty Lemon Herb Chicken and Rice to the soothing Vanilla Rice Pudding, each recipe is designed to be easy to follow and guaranteed to please both the palate and the body. Plus, with sections on how to stock your pantry and tips for maintaining a low histamine kitchen, this cookbook is also a mini-guide to embracing a low histamine lifestyle without sacrifice.

Whether you're a seasoned Instant Pot user or new to this type of cooking, the **Low Histamine Instant Pot Cookbook** will guide you through each step with clear instructions and plenty of tips to get the perfect results. It's about more than just meals; it's about making life simpler, healthier, and infinitely more delicious. Embrace the journey with confidence and creativity, and let your Instant Pot do the heavy lifting. Get ready to cook, enjoy, and thrive on your low histamine diet!

Chapter 1: Understanding Histamine

What Is Histamine?

Histamine is a naturally occurring compound that plays several important roles in the body, acting as a neurotransmitter, a component of the immune response, and a regulator of physiological functions in the gut. It's best known, however, for its involvement in the body's allergic responses and its role in conditions such as histamine intolerance.

Functions of Histamine
1. **Immune Response:** Histamine is part of the immune system's defense mechanism against foreign pathogens. When the body detects a harmful substance, immune cells release histamine as part of the inflammatory response. Histamine increases the permeability of the capillaries to white blood cells and some proteins, to allow them to engage pathogens in the infected tissues.
2. **Neurotransmitter:** As a neurotransmitter, histamine communicates important messages from the body to the brain. It is involved in several brain functions, including alertness, gastric secretion, and the sleep-wake cycle.
3. **Physiological Roles:** In the gut, histamine stimulates the secretion of gastric acid, aiding in digestion. It also plays a role in regulating physiological functions such as blood pressure, muscle contraction, and the dilation of blood vessels.

Histamine Intolerance
While histamine is essential for health, some individuals have difficulty breaking down and eliminating histamine from their bodies, leading to a condition known as histamine intolerance. This can result in an excess of histamine, which can cause various symptoms, including headaches, nasal congestion, fatigue, hives, digestive issues, and, in more severe cases, difficulty breathing.

Sources of Histamine

Histamine is found in various foods, especially those that are aged, fermented, or spoiled. Common high-histamine foods include aged cheeses, fermented foods (such as sauerkraut, kimchi, and soy products), alcohol (especially red wine and beer), and cured meats. The body also produces histamine naturally, and certain foods (even if not high in histamine themselves) can trigger the release of histamine from cells in the body.

Causes and Symptoms of Histamine Intolerance

Histamine intolerance is a condition where the body struggles to break down histamine efficiently, leading to an accumulation that can cause a range of symptoms. This imbalance is not an allergy itself but can lead to discomfort that mimics allergic reactions.

Causes of Histamine Intolerance
The primary cause of histamine intolerance is the body's inability to break down histamine properly, which is primarily due to deficiencies in an enzyme called diamine oxidase (DAO). This enzyme is responsible for breaking down histamine found in foods. When DAO levels are low or its activity is inhibited, histamine is not adequately metabolized, leading to increased histamine levels in the body. Several factors can contribute to this condition:
1. **Genetic Factors:** Some individuals may have a genetic predisposition that affects the production or activity of the DAO enzyme, making them more susceptible to histamine intolerance.
2. **Gastrointestinal Disorders:** Conditions such as inflammatory bowel disease (IBD), celiac disease, and Crohn's disease can damage the lining of the intestines where DAO is produced, leading to reduced enzyme levels and activity.
3. **Medications:** Certain medications can interfere with DAO function or histamine metabolism, including some pain relievers, antibiotics, antidepressants, and diuretics.
4. **Dietary Factors:** A diet high in histamine-rich foods can exacerbate symptoms of histamine intolerance, as it increases the overall histamine load that the body needs to process.
5. **Alcohol Consumption:** Alcohol can inhibit DAO activity and is also a source of histamine, both of which can worsen histamine intolerance symptoms.

Symptoms of Histamine Intolerance

Symptoms of histamine intolerance can vary widely among individuals and often mimic those of allergic reactions. They can be immediate or develop over time, making the condition challenging to diagnose. Common symptoms include:

1. **Skin Reactions:** Hives, eczema, or itchiness, particularly after consuming histamine-rich foods or alcoholic beverages.
2. **Digestive Symptoms:** Diarrhea, nausea, vomiting, and abdominal pain. These symptoms occur as histamine plays a role in gastric acid secretion and intestinal motility.
3. **Respiratory Issues:** Nasal congestion, sneezing, asthma, or difficulty breathing, which result from histamine-induced inflammation and swelling of airways.
4. **Neurological Symptoms:** Headaches, migraines, dizziness, or fatigue. Histamine acts as a neurotransmitter and can affect brain function.
5. **Cardiovascular Symptoms:** Flushing, rapid heartbeat, or hypotension, due to histamine-induced dilation of blood vessels.

Diagnosis and Management

Diagnosing histamine intolerance typically involves a detailed medical history, dietary review, and sometimes, the elimination of high-histamine foods followed by a controlled reintroduction. In some cases, blood tests for DAO activity or histamine levels may be helpful, though these are not always definitive.

Management strategies focus on reducing histamine exposure through dietary modifications, improving gut health to enhance DAO production, and using medications like antihistamines or DAO enzyme supplements to alleviate symptoms. Since histamine intolerance can overlap with other dietary sensitivities and health conditions, a holistic and personalized approach is often necessary for effective management.

Foods High in Histamine

Histamine intolerance can significantly affect individuals' quality of life, and dietary management is a critical component of controlling symptoms. Understanding which foods are high in histamine can help individuals tailor their diets to minimize discomfort. Histamine isn't uniformly distributed in foods; it accumulates in various amounts depending on the type of food, its storage, and how it's processed.

Fermented Foods
Fermentation is a process that can increase the histamine content in foods, as the microbial activity can produce histamine.
- **Sauerkraut:** A fermented cabbage known for its probiotic qualities but high in histamine.
- **Yogurt and Kefir:** While beneficial for gut health due to probiotics, some dairy products can be high in histamine.
- **Fermented soy products:** Including tempeh, soy sauce, and miso, which are staples in various cuisines but can be problematic for those with histamine intolerance.
- **Aged cheeses:** Such as cheddar, gouda, and blue cheese, have higher histamine levels due to the aging process.

Aged and Processed Meats
Aging and processing meats can increase their histamine content significantly.
- **Salami, pepperoni, and other cured meats:** The curing process involves fermentation, which increases histamine.
- **Aged hams** and **beef jerky** are also high in histamine due to the aging and drying processes.

Alcoholic Beverages
Alcohol and fermented beverages can both contain high levels of histamine and block the enzyme (DAO) that breaks down histamine in the body.
- **Red wine** and **beer** are particularly high in histamine, with white wine and some spirits generally being lower.

Seafood
Histamine levels in seafood can vary widely, often depending on the freshness of the product.
- **Fish, especially if not fresh or improperly stored:** Histamine can form rapidly in fish and seafood, making them potentially problematic.
- **Shellfish** also might have high levels of histamine, depending on freshness and processing.

Vegetables
While most vegetables are low in histamine, a few exceptions exist.
- **Tomatoes, spinach, and eggplant:** These can contain higher levels of histamine and also stimulate the body to release histamine.

Fruits
Certain fruits are known to contain histamine or trigger histamine release in the body.
- **Citrus fruits**, such as oranges, lemons, and grapefruits.
- **Strawberries** are also known to potentially trigger histamine release, though they are not high in histamine themselves.

Others
- **Chocolate**, **nuts**, and **foods containing artificial preservatives** and **colorings** can also have high histamine levels or trigger histamine release in the body.

Managing Histamine Intake
For those with histamine intolerance, managing dietary histamine can be challenging due to its presence in many nutritious foods. The key is identifying personal triggers, as tolerance levels can vary significantly between individuals. This often involves maintaining a food diary, eliminating high-histamine foods for a period, and then gradually reintroducing them to gauge tolerance. Working with a healthcare provider or a dietitian can provide personalized advice and support in managing histamine intolerance through diet. It's also worth noting that cooking methods and food freshness can impact histamine levels. Freshly cooked meals made from ingredients low in histamine tend to be better tolerated. Moreover, freezing fish immediately after catching can significantly reduce histamine formation, making certain types of seafood more manageable for those with histamine intolerance.

Foods Low in Histamine

Managing histamine intolerance effectively involves not only avoiding high-histamine foods but also focusing on those that are low in histamine. Incorporating low-histamine foods into the diet can help minimize symptoms and provide a balanced, nutritious intake without triggering histamine intolerance reactions. Here's an in-depth look at foods considered to be low in histamine, which can be safely included in the diet of those managing histamine levels.

Fresh Meats and Poultry
Freshly cooked meat and poultry are low in histamine. It's important that these foods are consumed soon after cooking, as histamine levels can increase with leftovers that are stored for a period.
- **Freshly cooked chicken, turkey, and lean cuts of beef:** Ensure they are consumed soon after cooking to avoid histamine buildup.

Freshly Caught Fish
While seafood is often high in histamine, especially if not fresh, certain practices can minimize histamine formation.
- **Freshly caught and immediately frozen fish:** This practice helps prevent the accumulation of histamine. Examples include freshly frozen salmon and trout.

Eggs
Eggs are a versatile and nutritious option that is naturally low in histamine, making them an excellent choice for all meals.

Dairy Substitutes
While aged cheeses and certain dairy products can be high in histamine, there are alternatives.
- **Fresh milk and dairy substitutes:** Such as coconut milk, almond milk, and rice milk, which are low in histamine.

Grains
Most grains are low in histamine, making them a safe staple for those with histamine intolerance.
- **Rice, oats, and quinoa:** These can be excellent bases for meals and are versatile in recipes.

Fresh Fruits
While some fruits can trigger histamine release, many are low in histamine and can be included in a low-histamine diet.
- **Apples, pears, and mangoes:** These fruits are typically well-tolerated.
- **Melons and kiwifruit:** Also low in histamine and good options for a sweet treat.

Vegetables
Most vegetables are low in histamine, though it's important to avoid those known to trigger histamine release.
- **Leafy greens (excluding spinach), carrots, and potatoes:** These are nutritious and versatile.
- **Broccoli, squash, and cucumbers:** These vegetables are also safe and can be included in a variety of dishes.

Cooking Oils and Fats
The right kinds of fats are essential for a balanced diet and most are low in histamine.
- **Olive oil and coconut oil:** These are excellent choices for cooking and preparing food.

Herbs and Spices
Most fresh herbs and some spices are low in histamine, though it's important to use them fresh and avoid mixes that might contain additives.
- **Basil, oregano, and thyme:** Fresh herbs can add flavor to dishes without adding histamine.

Beverages

Choosing the right beverages is crucial in managing histamine levels.

- **Fresh water, herbal teas, and certain non-caffeinated drinks:** These are safe choices. It's important to avoid alcohol and fermented beverages, which are high in histamine.

Managing a Low-Histamine Diet

When managing histamine intolerance, the freshness of the food is key. Histamine levels can increase in foods over time, especially if they are stored improperly. Thus, it's essential to consume fresh foods and prepare meals at home whenever possible. Moreover, individual reactions to histamine can vary, so keeping a food diary to track symptoms in response to different foods can be helpful in identifying personal triggers.

Chapter 2: Understanding Your Instant Pot

What is an Instant Pot?
The Instant Pot combines several kitchen appliances into one. It can function as a pressure cooker, slow cooker, rice cooker, steamer, sauté pan, yogurt maker, and warmer. This versatility not only saves kitchen space but also makes meal preparation quicker and more convenient.

Key Components and Their Functions
- **Inner Pot:** This is the removable container where all the cooking happens. It's usually made of stainless steel, making it durable and easy to clean.
- **Lid:** The lid locks in place during cooking, creating a sealed environment that allows pressure to build. It has a sealing ring to prevent steam from escaping and a valve that controls the release of pressure.
- **Control Panel:** Depending on your model, the control panel may have buttons or a digital touch screen. Here, you select cooking modes, adjust times, and set pressures. Familiarizing yourself with these controls is key to mastering your Instant Pot.
- **Pressure Release Valve:** This critical safety feature allows you to manually release pressure from the pot. Understanding when and how to use it is crucial for safety and cooking success.

Safety Features
The Instant Pot is equipped with numerous safety features designed to prevent common pressure cooking accidents. These include a lid lock under pressure, overpressure and temperature controls, and automatic pressure control. These features make the Instant Pot safer to use than traditional pressure cookers.

Getting Started: The Water Test
Performing a water test is a recommended first step for new Instant Pot users. This simple procedure involves adding water to the pot and running a short pressure cycle. It's a way to ensure your Instant Pot is functioning correctly and gives you a risk-free opportunity to familiarize yourself with its basic operations.

Essential Accessories

While the Instant Pot comes equipped with the basic necessities for pressure cooking, a multitude of additional accessories can elevate your cooking experience, making your culinary creations more diverse and your kitchen routines smoother. Here's a rundown of some essential and highly recommended accessories for any Instant Pot user:

1. Steamer Basket
A steamer basket is crucial for anyone looking to use their Instant Pot for steaming vegetables, fish, or even making hard-boiled eggs. It's designed to keep food items above the water level, allowing them to steam perfectly. Silicone or metal options are available, with some models featuring handles for easy removal.

2. Extra Sealing Rings
The silicone sealing ring in the lid is key to keeping the Instant Pot airtight and safe. Over time, these rings can absorb odors or become worn. Having extra sealing rings on hand, possibly even designated ones for sweet and savory dishes, ensures your Instant Pot is always ready for action without transferring flavors.

3. Glass Lid
A glass lid is perfect for when you're using the Instant Pot as a slow cooker or when you're keeping food warm. It allows you to see inside the pot without lifting the lid, helping to retain heat and moisture. This accessory is essential for dishes that benefit from slow cooking or any time you need to check progress without releasing steam.

4. Springform Pan or Push Pan
For those interested in baking in their Instant Pot, a springform pan or push pan that fits inside the pot is a must-have. These pans are ideal for making cheesecakes, lasagnas, or even bread. They make it easy to prepare and remove delicate dishes without them falling apart.

5. Silicone Egg Bites Mold
Popular among Instant Pot enthusiasts, silicone egg bites molds are great for making egg bites, mini cheesecakes, or baby food. They offer a convenient and easy way to prepare bite-sized treats or breakfast options that are perfectly portioned and easily customizable.

6. Stackable Insert Pans
For those looking to maximize their Instant Pot's efficiency, stackable insert pans allow you to cook multiple dishes at once, such as rice in one pan and chicken in another. This accessory is a game-changer for meal prep or when preparing multi-component meals.

7. Silicone Mitts or Grips
Handling the inner pot or accessories when hot can be challenging. Silicone mitts or grips designed for the Instant Pot provide a safe way to handle hot components, making the cooking process safer and more comfortable.

8. Trivet with Handles
While a basic trivet likely comes with your Instant Pot, versions with handles make it easier to lift dishes, pans, or steamer baskets out of the pot, especially when they're hot. It's particularly useful for dishes like whole chickens or large cuts of meat.

9. Cheesecake Push Pan
A push pan is similar to a springform pan but uses a different mechanism to release the cake. It's incredibly useful for making not just cheesecakes but also other desserts and dishes that need to be unmolded from a pan.

Investing in these accessories can significantly enhance your Instant Pot experience, making it more versatile and convenient. Whether you're a new user or looking to expand your cooking repertoire, incorporating a few or all of these accessories into your kitchen can open up a world of culinary possibilities, from steaming and baking to multi-dish preparation, all with the ease and speed the Instant Pot is famous for.

Common Terms and Functions

Common Terms
- **Pressure Cooking:** This is the process of cooking food at high pressure, which significantly reduces cooking time while preserving nutrients and flavors. The Instant Pot uses steam pressure built up inside the sealed pot to cook food efficiently.
- **Natural Pressure Release (NPR):** After the cooking cycle finishes, the Instant Pot naturally decreases pressure over time without any intervention. This process can take anywhere from 10 to 30 minutes, depending on the volume and type of food. It's ideal for foods that benefit from a longer cooking time, like meats and stews, to prevent them from becoming tough.
- **Quick Release (QR):** This method involves manually turning the steam release valve to the venting position to let the steam escape quickly, stopping the cooking process immediately. It's used for delicate items like vegetables or seafood that might overcook if left in too long.
- **Sauté:** The Instant Pot can heat and simmer food without the lid, similar to a traditional stovetop pan. This function is great for browning meat, softening vegetables, or thickening sauces before pressure cooking.
- **Sealing Ring:** A silicone gasket that ensures the lid is airtight and steam doesn't escape during pressure cooking. It's crucial for the safety and efficiency of the Instant Pot.
- **Steam Release Valve:** Located on the lid, this valve controls the release of steam and pressure. It must be set to the sealing position for pressure cooking and can be manually opened for quick pressure release.

Key Functions

- **Manual/Pressure Cook:** This is the basic function that lets you set the cooking time at high or low pressure. It's the most commonly used feature for recipes not specific to any other preset cooking program.
- **Rice:** Automatically adjusts the cooking time for white rice, providing perfectly cooked grains every time. It's specifically designed for cooking rice and should not be used for other types of grains or recipes.
- **Multigrain:** This setting is for cooking hearty grains like brown rice, wild rice, or other mixes that require a longer cooking time than white rice.
- **Soup/Broth:** Optimized for making soups and broths, this function cooks at a lower pressure to prevent rapid boiling, ensuring clear broths and intact ingredients.
- **Meat/Stew:** Ideal for cooking meat and stews, this setting increases the cooking time to tenderize meats and blend flavors thoroughly.
- **Bean/Chili:** This function is tailored for cooking beans and legumes, whether soaked or unsoaked, ensuring they're perfectly cooked without presoaking.
- **Yogurt:** A unique feature of the Instant Pot that allows you to ferment milk into yogurt. It maintains a consistent low temperature over several hours, essential for the fermentation process.
- **Slow Cook:** Mimics a traditional slow cooker, allowing you to cook recipes at a lower temperature for several hours. The Instant Pot can be set to different heat settings (low, medium, high) similar to a standard slow cooker.

Understanding these terms and functions is the first step towards becoming an Instant Pot pro. Each function is designed to make specific cooking tasks easier and more intuitive, allowing you to explore a wide range of recipes with confidence. As you become more familiar with these features, you'll find that the Instant Pot can be an invaluable tool in your kitchen, saving you time and expanding your culinary capabilities.

Tips for Successful Instant Pot Cooking

Successful Instant Pot cooking is about more than just throwing ingredients into the pot and hoping for the best. It requires understanding the nuances of how pressure cooking works, what the Instant Pot excels at, and the small but significant details that can transform a good dish into a great one. Here are some thorough pointers for becoming an Instant Pot cooking expert:

1. **Read the Manual**
   - Before diving into recipes, thoroughly read your Instant Pot's manual. Each model has its quirks, and understanding the basic operations, safety features, and maintenance requirements is crucial for both safety and cooking success.

2. **Understand Liquid Requirements**
   - The Instant Pot needs liquid to generate steam for pressure cooking. Most recipes require at least 1 cup of liquid, but always refer to your manual for the minimum amount your specific model requires. Too little liquid can lead to burned food or a malfunctioning pot.

3. **Use Natural vs. Quick Release Wisely**
   - Know when to use natural pressure release (NPR) and when to use quick release (QR). NPR is best for dense, starchy foods and large cuts of meat, as it prevents sputtering and allows for continued cooking as the pot naturally depressurizes. QR is suitable for delicate items like vegetables, preventing them from overcooking.

4. **Don't Overfill the Pot**
   - Respect the max-fill lines inside your Instant Pot. Overfilling, especially with foods that expand (like grains or beans) or foam (like pasta), can clog the vent pipe and affect cooking performance or safety.

5. **Sauté Before Pressure Cooking**
   - Utilize the sauté function to brown meats or soften vegetables before pressure cooking. This step adds depth of flavor to dishes and can help reduce cooking liquids for richer sauces.

6. Deglaze the Pot
- After sautéing, pour a bit of liquid into the pot and scrape up any browned bits from the bottom. This technique, known as deglazing, not only incorporates more flavor into your dish but also prevents the "Burn" error by cleaning the pot bottom.

7. Layer Ingredients Strategically
- Place ingredients that take longer to cook at the bottom, closer to the heat source. Add delicate ingredients on top or add them after pressure cooking through a technique called "Pot in Pot" (placing another container inside the Instant Pot) when necessary.

8. Seal Correctly
- Ensure the sealing ring is properly positioned and the steam release valve is set to "Sealing." A misplaced sealing ring or an incorrectly set valve is a common reason for cooking failures.

9. Embrace Water Test
- Perform the water test (outlined in the manual) before your first use. It's a simple way to ensure your Instant Pot is working correctly and familiarize yourself with the pressure cooking process.

10. Adjust Recipes for Altitude
- If you live at a high altitude, adjust your cooking time. Pressure cooking times increase slightly at higher elevations due to lower atmospheric pressure. A general rule is to increase cooking time by 5% for every 1,000 feet above 2,000 feet elevation.

11. Experiment and Be Patient
- Instant Pot cooking is as much an art as it is a science. Not every recipe will be perfect on the first try. Be patient, adjust as necessary, and don't be afraid to experiment. Learning the nuances of your particular Instant Pot model will come with time and experience.

Why Use an Instant Pot for Your Low Histamine Diet?

1. Speed and Convenience
The Instant Pot is renowned for its ability to cook meals faster than traditional methods, thanks to its pressure cooking feature. This speed is a boon for those on a low histamine diet, as fresh foods are a staple and it's essential to prepare meals quickly to minimize histamine formation, which can increase over time in cooked and stored foods.

2. Preserving Nutrients
Cooking with an Instant Pot can help preserve the vitamins and minerals in your food. Because the cooking time is shorter and often uses less water than traditional cooking methods, fewer nutrients are lost during the cooking process. This is especially important for a low histamine diet, where maximizing the nutritional value of each meal can support overall health and help manage histamine intolerance symptoms.

3. Versatility
The Instant Pot's versatility means you can use it for a wide range of dishes, from breakfasts to desserts, all in one pot. This can include steaming vegetables, cooking grains, making stews, and even yogurt – all of which are staples in a low histamine diet. This versatility also reduces the need for multiple cooking appliances, saving space in the kitchen and reducing cleanup time.

4. Reduced Histamine Build-Up
Since the Instant Pot cooks meals quickly and efficiently, it can help in reducing the time food is exposed to air and warmth, conditions under which histamines can develop. Cooking fresh meals quickly and consuming them immediately can be an effective strategy in managing a low histamine diet.

5. Contamination Control
Using an Instant Pot can also help in reducing cross-contamination with high-histamine foods. Since everything is cooked in one pot, there's less likelihood of mixing utensils or cookware that might have residues of high-histamine ingredients. This can be particularly beneficial for individuals who are highly sensitive to dietary histamines.

6. Batch Cooking
The Instant Pot is ideal for batch cooking, which is convenient for those on a strict diet. Preparing large quantities of low histamine meals ahead of time can be a timesaver. The Instant Pot's keep-warm function also means food can be kept at a safe temperature until ready to eat, without significantly increasing histamine levels.

7. Ease of Use
Finally, the simplicity of using an Instant Pot – with its set-and-forget functionality – makes it accessible even to those who may not be very experienced in the kitchen. This ease of use encourages cooking at home, an essential aspect of following a low histamine diet, where control over ingredients and cooking methods is crucial.

BREAKFAST

1. Quinoa Apple Cinnamon Breakfast Bowl
Ingredients:
- 1 cup quinoa (rinsed)
- 2 cups water
- 2 medium apples, peeled and diced
- 1 teaspoon cinnamon
- A pinch of salt
- Optional toppings: maple syrup, chopped nuts (ensure low histamine)

Instructions:
1. Combine the rinsed quinoa, water, diced apples, cinnamon, and a pinch of salt in the Instant Pot.
2. Secure the lid, setting the valve to the sealing position. Select the "Manual" or "Pressure Cook" setting, and set the timer for 1 minute at high pressure. The quinoa cooks quickly, and the Instant Pot will take about 10 minutes to reach pressure before the cooking time begins.
3. After the cooking cycle completes, allow the Instant Pot to naturally release pressure for about 10 minutes, then carefully do a quick release for any remaining steam.
4. Open the lid, stir the quinoa and apple mixture, and serve warm with optional toppings as desired.

Nutrition Info (Per Serving, without toppings):
Calories: 235 Protein: 8g Fat: 3.5g Carbohydrates: 45g Fiber: 5g
- Serving Size: 4 servings
- Cooking Time: Approximately 20 minutes (including pressure build-up and release)

2. Pear and Cardamom Steel-cut Oats

Ingredients:
- 1 cup steel-cut oats
- 2 cups water
- 2 ripe pears, peeled and chopped
- 1 teaspoon ground cardamom
- A pinch of salt
- Optional toppings: sliced almonds, a drizzle of honey (if tolerated)

Instructions:
1. Add the steel-cut oats, water, chopped pears, ground cardamom, and a pinch of salt to the Instant Pot. Stir to combine.
2. Place the lid on the Instant Pot, ensuring the valve is set to the sealing position. Select "Manual" or "Pressure Cook" and set the time for 4 minutes on high pressure. It will take the Instant Pot approximately 10-15 minutes to reach pressure.
3. After the cooking cycle is complete, allow the Instant Pot to naturally release pressure for about 10 minutes, then carefully perform a quick release for any remaining steam.
4. Open the lid once it's safe to do so, stir the oats, and adjust the seasoning if necessary. Serve warm with optional toppings.

Nutrition Info (Per Serving, without toppings):
- Calories: 150
- Protein: 5g
- Fat: 2.5g
- Carbohydrates: 27g
- Fiber: 4g
- Serving Size: 4 servings
- Cooking Time: Approximately 25 minutes (including pressure build-up and release)

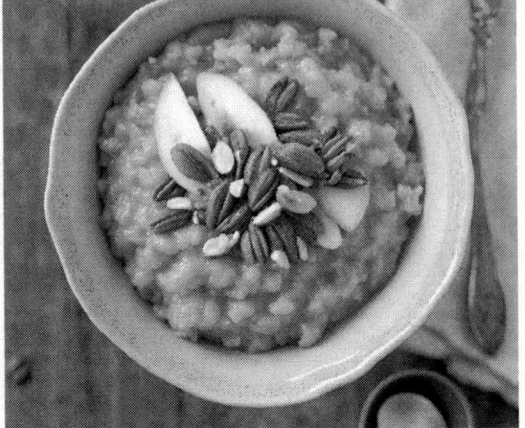

3. Coconut Rice Pudding

Ingredients:
- 1 cup Arborio rice (or any other short-grain white rice)
- 1 can (13.5 oz) coconut milk
- 2 cups water
- 1/4 cup sugar (adjust to taste)
- 1/2 teaspoon vanilla extract
- A pinch of salt

Instructions:
1. Rinse the rice under cold water until the water runs clear.
2. Combine the rinsed rice, coconut milk, water, sugar, vanilla extract, and a pinch of salt in the Instant Pot.
3. Stir to mix everything thoroughly.
4. Secure the lid, turn the valve to sealing, and set the Instant Pot to cook on High Pressure for 20 minutes.
5. Once the cooking is complete, allow the pot to naturally release pressure for 10 minutes, then carefully perform a quick release for any remaining pressure.
6. Stir the rice pudding before serving to blend all ingredients well.

Nutrition Info (Per Serving):
- Calories: 280
- Protein: 3g
- Fat: 12g
- Carbohydrates: 40g
- Fiber: 0g
- Serving Size: 6 servings
- Cooking Time: 30 minutes total

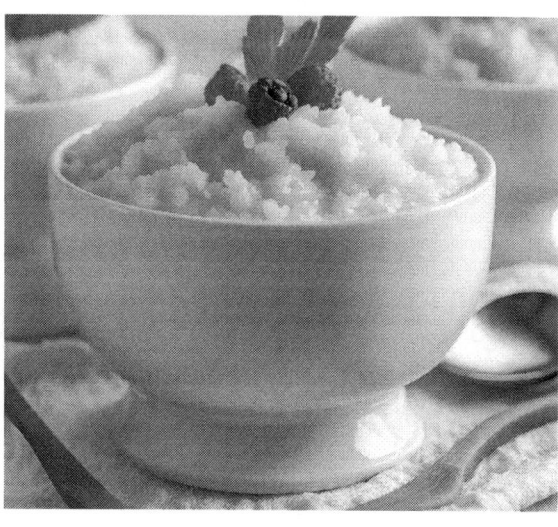

4. Ginger-infused Millet Porridge

Ingredients:
- 1 cup millet, rinsed
- 3 cups water
- 1 tablespoon freshly grated ginger
- A pinch of salt

Instructions:
1. Add rinsed millet, water, grated ginger, and a pinch of salt to the Instant Pot.
2. Stir to combine.
3. Close the lid, set the valve to sealing, and cook on High Pressure for 10 minutes.
4. Let the Instant Pot naturally release pressure for 10 minutes, then do a quick release for any remaining steam.
5. Stir the porridge well before serving; it should be creamy and thick.

Nutrition Info (Per Serving):
- Calories: 200
- Protein: 6g
- Fat: 2g
- Carbohydrates: 39g
- Fiber: 2g
- Serving Size: 4 servings
- Cooking Time: 20 minutes total

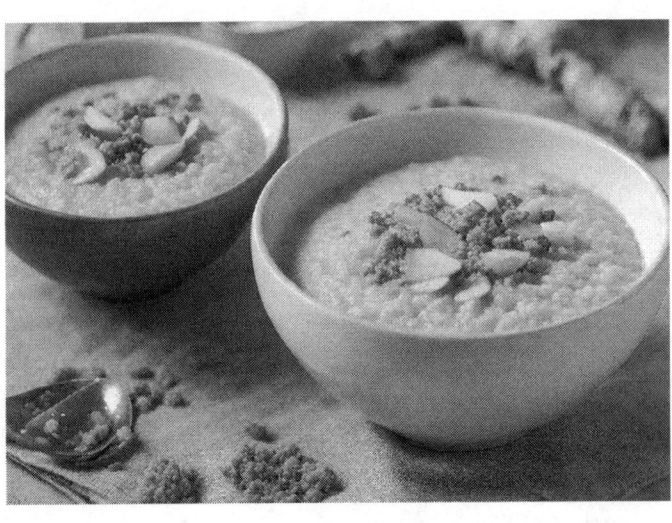

5. Vegetable Frittata

Ingredients:
- 8 eggs
- 1/2 cup milk (or dairy-free alternative)
- 1 cup chopped spinach
- 1/2 cup diced bell peppers
- 1/4 cup diced onions
- Salt and pepper to taste
- 1 tablespoon olive oil

Instructions:
1. In a bowl, whisk together eggs, milk, spinach, bell peppers, onions, salt, and pepper.
2. Turn the Instant Pot to sauté mode and heat the olive oil.
3. Pour the egg mixture into the pot once hot.
4. Cancel the sauté function, close the lid, set the valve to sealing, and set the Instant Pot on High Pressure for 5 minutes.
5. Quick release the pressure immediately after the cooking time is over.
6. Serve the frittata directly from the pot or inverted onto a plate.

Nutrition Info (Per Serving):
- Calories: 160
- Protein: 10g
- Fat: 12g
- Carbohydrates: 3g
- Fiber: 1g
- Serving Size: 6 servings
- Cooking Time: 15 minutes total

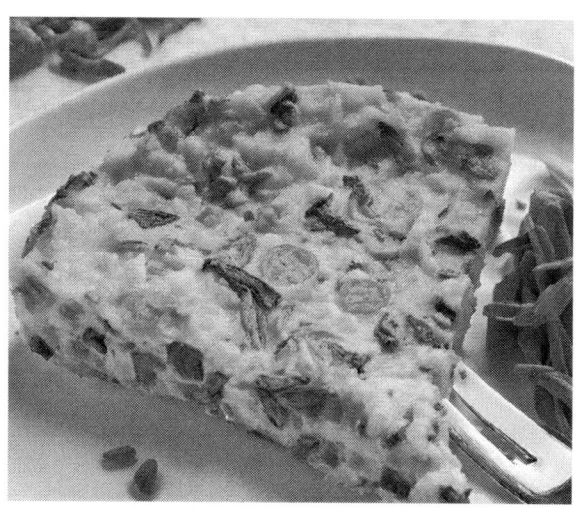

6. Jumbo Blueberry Pancake

Ingredients:
- 1 cup all-purpose flour
- 1 tablespoon sugar
- 1 teaspoon baking powder
- 1/2 teaspoon salt
- 3/4 cup milk
- 1 egg
- 2 tablespoons melted butter
- 1/2 cup blueberries

Instructions:
1. In a bowl, mix flour, sugar, baking powder, and salt.
2. Whisk in milk, egg, and melted butter until the batter is smooth.
3. Fold in the blueberries gently.
4. Pour the batter into a greased cake pan that fits in your Instant Pot.
5. Pour 1 cup of water into the bottom of the Instant Pot, place the trivet, and set the cake pan on top of the trivet.
6. Close the lid, set the valve to sealing, and use the Manual setting to cook for 15 minutes on High Pressure.
7. Let the pressure release naturally for 10 minutes, then do a quick release.
8. Serve the pancake warm.

Nutrition Info (Per Serving):
- Calories: 180
- Protein: 4g
- Fat: 6g
- Carbohydrates: 27g
- Fiber: 1g
- Serving Size: 4 servings
- Cooking Time: 25minutes

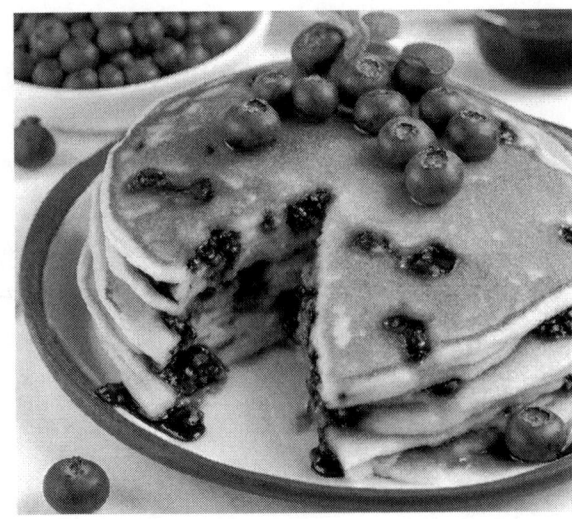

7. Buckwheat Banana Pancakes

Ingredients:
- 1 cup buckwheat flour
- 1 teaspoon baking powder
- 1/4 teaspoon salt
- 1 ripe banana, mashed
- 1 cup milk
- 1 egg
- 2 tablespoons melted coconut oil

Instructions:
1. Combine buckwheat flour, baking powder, and salt in a large mixing bowl.
2. In another bowl, mix the mashed banana, milk, egg, and melted coconut oil.
3. Add the wet ingredients to the dry ingredients and stir until just combined.
4. Pour the batter into a greased cake pan suitable for the Instant Pot.
5. Add 1 cup of water to the pot, place the trivet, and set the pan on the trivet.
6. Close the lid, set the valve to sealing, and cook on High Pressure for 15 minutes.
7. Allow natural pressure release for 10 minutes, followed by a quick release.
8. Serve the pancakes warm.

Nutrition Info (Per Serving):
- Calories: 210
- Protein: 5g
- Fat: 9g
- Carbohydrates: 29g
- Fiber: 3g
- Serving Size: 4 servings
- Cooking Time: 25 minutes total

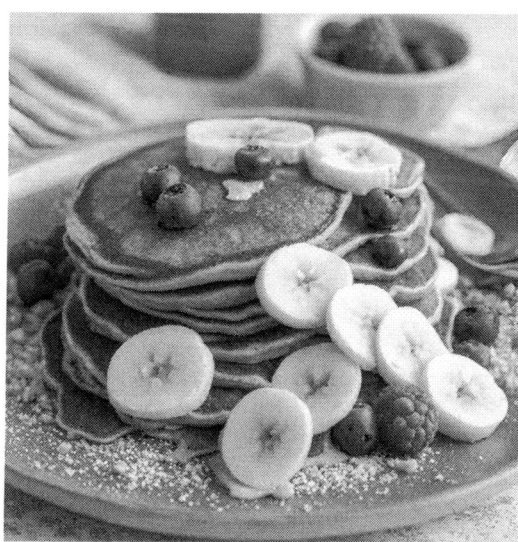

8. Savory Chicken and Rice Congee

Ingredients:
- 1 cup jasmine rice
- 6 cups low sodium chicken broth
- 2 boneless skinless chicken thighs
- 1 teaspoon salt
- 1 inch ginger, finely chopped
- Optional garnishes: chopped green onions, a drizzle of sesame oil

Instructions:
1. Rinse jasmine rice under cold water until the water runs clear.
2. Combine rice, chicken broth, chicken thighs, salt, and ginger in the Instant Pot.
3. Secure the lid, set the valve to sealing, and cook on the Porridge setting for 20 minutes.
4. Allow the pressure to naturally release for 15 minutes, then manually release any remaining pressure.
5. Open the lid, remove the chicken thighs, shred them, and return the shredded chicken to the pot.
6. Stir well and serve hot with optional garnishes.

Nutrition Info (Per Serving):
- Calories: 225
- Protein: 18g
- Fat: 3g
- Carbohydrates: 33g
- Fiber: 1g
- Serving Size: 6 servings
- Cooking Time: 35 minutes total

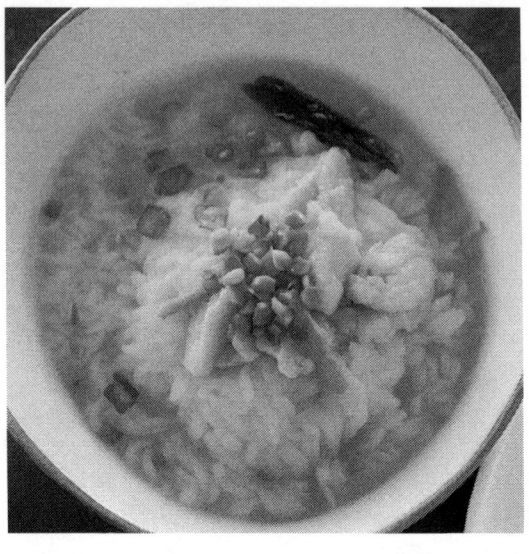

9. Sweet Potato and Kale Hash

Ingredients:
- 2 large sweet potatoes, peeled and diced
- 1 bunch kale, stems removed and leaves chopped
- 1 onion, chopped
- 2 tablespoons olive oil
- Salt and pepper to taste

Instructions:
1. Set the Instant Pot to sauté mode and heat the olive oil.
2. Add the chopped onion and sauté until translucent.
3. Add diced sweet potatoes, chopped kale, salt, and pepper, and stir to combine.
4. Add 1/4 cup water to prevent burning and cancel sauté mode.
5. Close the lid, set the valve to sealing, and cook on Manual High Pressure for 4 minutes.
6. Quick release the pressure once cooking is complete.
7. Open the lid and stir the hash before serving.

Nutrition Info (Per Serving):
- Calories: 160
- Protein: 3g
- Fat: 7g
- Carbohydrates: 23g
- Fiber: 4g
- Serving Size: 4 servings
- Cooking Time: 20 minutes total

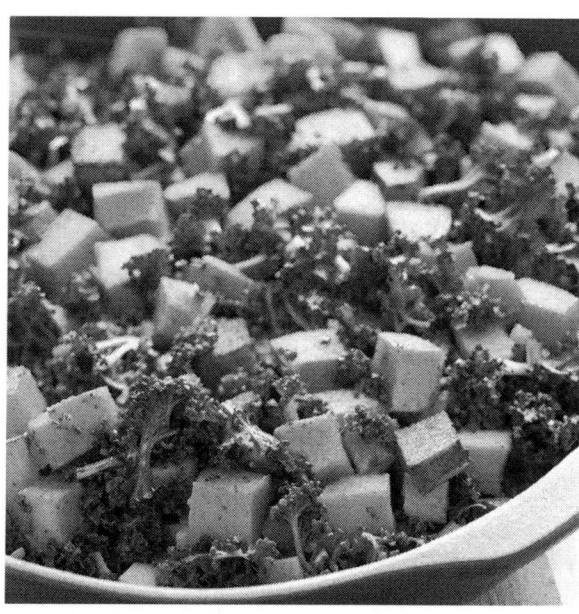

10. Mango Coconut Chia Pudding

Ingredients:
- 1 cup coconut milk
- 1/4 cup chia seeds
- 1 mango, peeled and diced
- 2 tablespoons honey (optional, adjust according to histamine tolerance)
- 1/2 teaspoon vanilla extract

Instructions:
1. In a bowl, mix together coconut milk, chia seeds, honey, and vanilla extract.
2. Stir in the diced mango.
3. Pour the mixture into a container that can fit inside the Instant Pot.
4. Pour 1 cup of water into the Instant Pot and place the trivet inside.
5. Set the container on the trivet, close the lid, and set the valve to sealing.
6. Use the Steam setting for 2 minutes.
7. Allow natural pressure release for 10 minutes, then remove the pudding and chill before serving.

Nutrition Info (Per Serving):
- Calories: 215
- Protein: 3g
- Fat: 15g
- Carbohydrates: 19g
- Fiber: 5g
- Serving Size: 4 servings
- Cooking Time: 12 minutes total

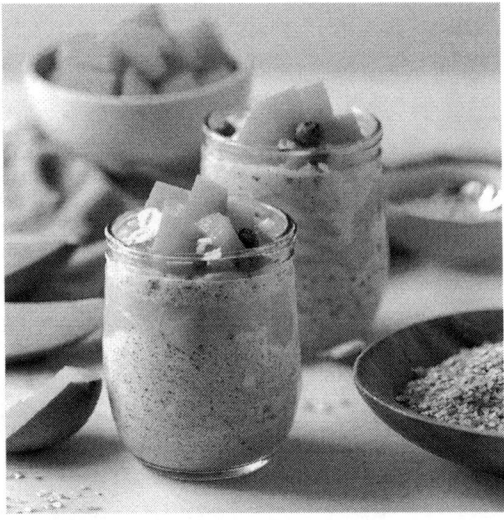

11. Apple and Walnut Breakfast Quinoa

Ingredients:
- 1 cup quinoa, rinsed
- 2 cups water
- 2 apples, diced
- 1/2 cup walnuts, chopped
- 1 teaspoon cinnamon
- 2 tablespoons honey (optional)

Instructions:
1. Add quinoa, water, diced apples, cinnamon, and honey to the Instant Pot.
2. Stir to combine and then secure the lid, setting the valve to sealing.
3. Cook on Manual High Pressure for 1 minute.
4. Allow the pressure to naturally release for 10 minutes, then quick release any remaining pressure.
5. Stir in chopped walnuts before serving.

Nutrition Info (Per Serving):
- Calories: 320
- Protein: 8g
- Fat: 10g
- Carbohydrates: 53g
- Fiber: 6g
- Serving Size: 4 servings
- Cooking Time: 11 minutes total

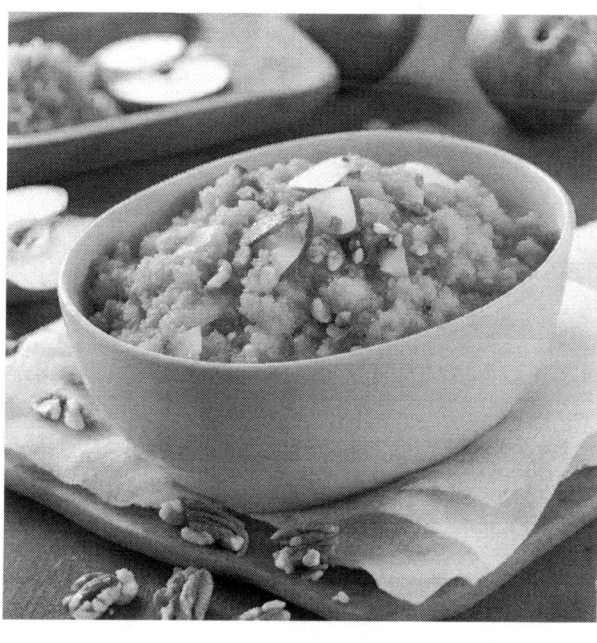

12. Pumpkin Spice Oatmeal

Ingredients:
- 1 cup steel-cut oats
- 3 cups water
- 1 cup pumpkin puree
- 1 teaspoon cinnamon
- 1/2 teaspoon nutmeg
- 1/4 teaspoon cloves
- 2 tablespoons maple syrup (optional)

Instructions:
1. Add all ingredients to the Instant Pot and stir to combine.
2. Close the lid, set the valve to sealing, and cook on Manual High Pressure for 4 minutes.
3. Allow the pressure to naturally release for 10 minutes, then quick release any remaining pressure.
4. Stir the oatmeal well before serving.

Nutrition Info (Per Serving):
- Calories: 200
- Protein: 6g
- Fat: 3g
- Carbohydrates: 38g
- Fiber: 6g
- Serving Size: 4 servings
- Cooking Time: 14 minutes total

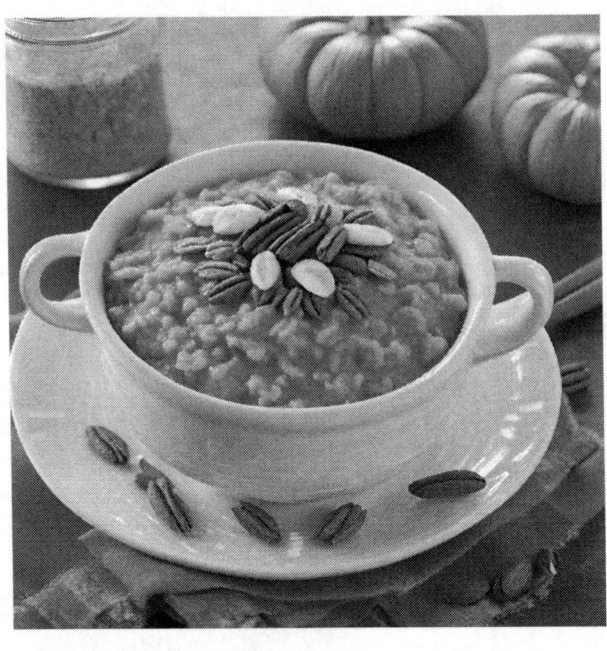

13. Lemon and Herb Quinoa Breakfast Pilaf

Ingredients:
- 1 cup quinoa, rinsed
- 2 cups vegetable broth
- Juice and zest of 1 lemon
- 1 tablespoon olive oil
- 1/4 cup chopped parsley
- 1 teaspoon thyme
- Salt and pepper to taste

Instructions:
1. Add quinoa, vegetable broth, lemon juice, zest, olive oil, and thyme to the Instant Pot.
2. Stir to combine, close the lid, and set the valve to sealing.
3. Cook on Manual High Pressure for 1 minute.
4. Allow natural pressure release for 10 minutes, then quick release any remaining pressure.
5. Stir in chopped parsley and season with salt and pepper before serving.

Nutrition Info (Per Serving):
- Calories: 222
- Protein: 8g
- Fat: 6g
- Carbohydrates: 35g
- Fiber: 4g
- Serving Size: 4 servings
- Cooking Time: 11 minutes total

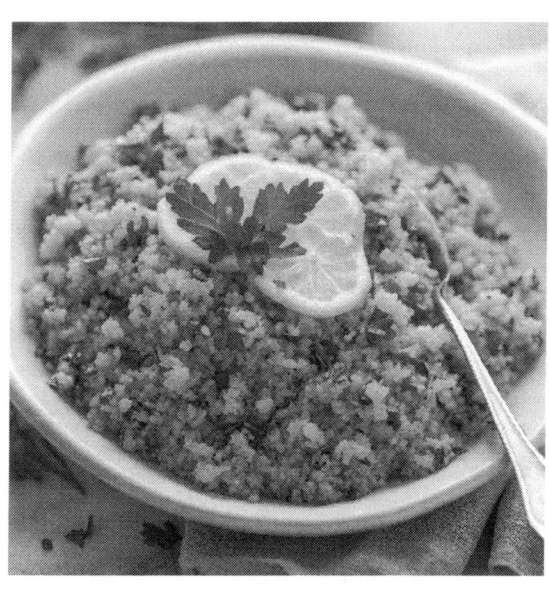

14. Instant Pot Poached Pears

Ingredients:
- 4 pears, peeled, halved, and cored
- 1 cup water
- 1/2 cup honey
- 2 cinnamon sticks
- 4 cloves

Instructions:
1. Place water, honey, cinnamon sticks, and cloves into the Instant Pot and stir to combine.
2. Add the pear halves to the pot.
3. Secure the lid, set the valve to sealing, and cook on Manual High Pressure for 3 minutes.
4. Allow the pressure to naturally release for 10 minutes, then quick release any remaining pressure.
5. Serve the pears warm with some of the cooking liquid drizzled over them.

Nutrition Info (Per Serving):
- Calories: 160
- Protein: 0g
- Fat: 0g
- Carbohydrates: 42g
- Fiber: 6g
- Serving Size: 4 servings
- Cooking Time: 13 minutes total

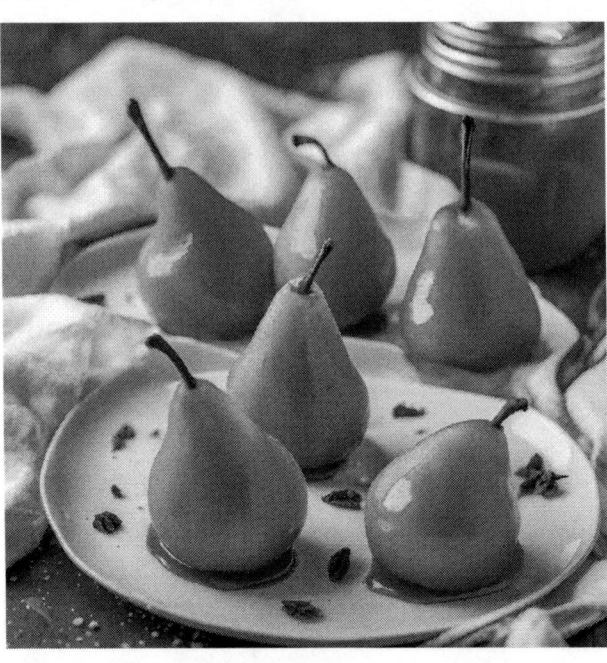

15. Turkey and Sweet Potato Breakfast Casserole

Ingredients:
- 1 pound ground turkey
- 2 sweet potatoes, peeled and grated
- 1 onion, diced
- 1 bell pepper, diced
- 12 eggs, beaten
- 1 teaspoon salt
- 1/2 teaspoon black pepper

Instructions:
1. Set the Instant Pot to sauté mode and brown the ground turkey with the diced onion and bell pepper.
2. Add the grated sweet potatoes and stir to mix.
3. Pour the beaten eggs over the turkey and vegetable mixture. Do not stir.
4. Secure the lid, set the valve to sealing, and cook on Manual High Pressure for 15 minutes.
5. Quick release the pressure after cooking.
6. Serve the casserole directly from the pot.

Nutrition Info (Per Serving):
- Calories: 320
- Protein: 28g
- Fat: 18g
- Carbohydrates: 12g
- Fiber: 2g
- Serving Size: 6 servings
- Cooking Time: 30 minutes total

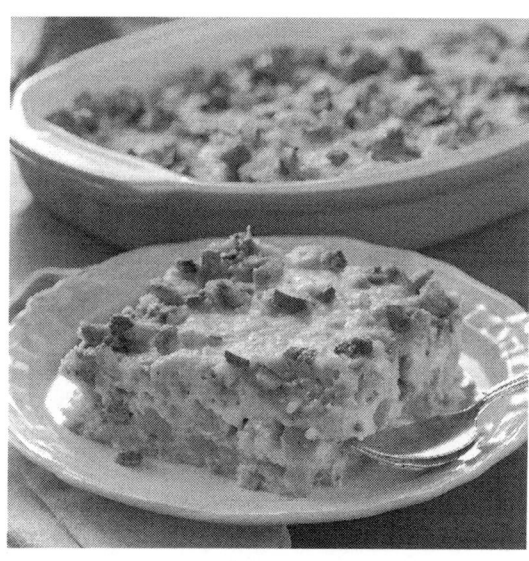

16. Zucchini and Carrot Breakfast Muffins

Ingredients:
- 1 cup grated zucchini
- 1 cup grated carrot
- 1 1/2 cups almond flour
- 1/4 cup olive oil
- 3 eggs
- 1 teaspoon baking powder
- 1/2 teaspoon salt

Instructions:
1. In a large bowl, mix together grated zucchini, carrot, almond flour, olive oil, eggs, baking powder, and salt until well combined.
2. Divide the mixture into silicone muffin cups.
3. Pour 1 cup of water into the Instant Pot and place the trivet inside.
4. Arrange the muffin cups on the trivet.
5. Close the lid, set the valve to sealing, and cook on Manual High Pressure for 15 minutes.
6. Let the pressure naturally release for 10 minutes, then quick release any remaining pressure.
7. Carefully remove the muffins and let them cool before serving.

Nutrition Info (Per Serving):
- Calories: 220
- Protein: 7g
- Fat: 18g
- Carbohydrates: 8g
- Fiber: 3g
- Serving Size: 6 servings
- Cooking Time: 25 minutes total

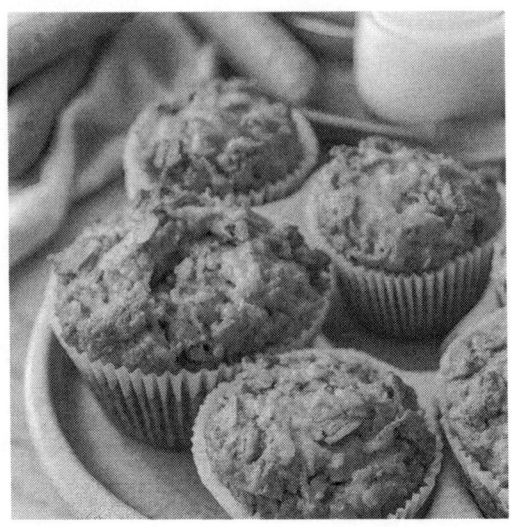

17. Blueberry Millet Porridge

Ingredients:
- 1 cup millet, rinsed
- 3 cups water
- 1 cup blueberries
- 1/2 teaspoon cinnamon
- 1 tablespoon honey (optional)

Instructions:
1. Add millet, water, blueberries, and cinnamon to the Instant Pot. Drizzle honey over the top if using.
2. Stir to mix all ingredients.
3. Secure the lid, set the valve to sealing, and cook on Manual High Pressure for 10 minutes.
4. Allow the pressure to naturally release for 10 minutes, then quick release any remaining pressure.
5. Stir the porridge well before serving.

Nutrition Info (Per Serving):
- Calories: 215
- Protein: 6g
- Fat: 2g
- Carbohydrates: 45g
- Fiber: 4g
- Serving Size: 4 servings
- Cooking Time: 20 minutes total

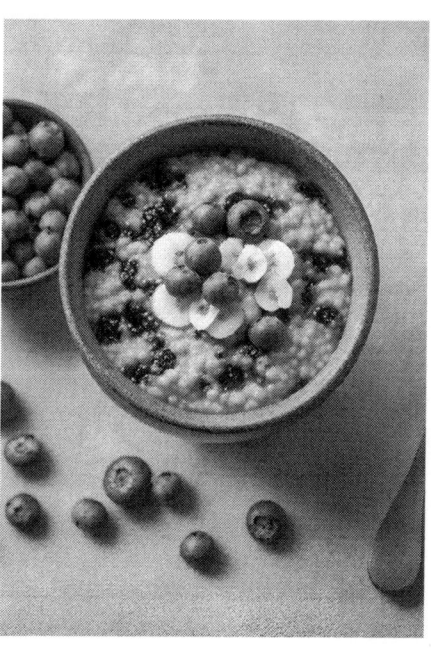

18. Spinach and Potato Breakfast Frittata

Ingredients:
- 6 eggs
- 1 cup chopped spinach
- 1 large potato, diced
- 1 onion, diced
- 1/2 cup milk
- Salt and pepper to taste
- 1 tablespoon olive oil

Instructions:
1. Set the Instant Pot to sauté mode and heat the olive oil.
2. Add the diced potato and onion and sauté until the onion is translucent.
3. Stir in the chopped spinach and sauté for another minute.
4. In a bowl, whisk together eggs, milk, salt, and pepper.
5. Pour the egg mixture over the sautéed vegetables.
6. Cancel the sauté mode, close the lid, set the valve to sealing, and cook on Manual High Pressure for 5 minutes.
7. Quick release the pressure immediately after the cooking time is over.
8. Serve the frittata directly from the pot.

Nutrition Info (Per Serving):
- Calories: 180
- Protein: 10g
- Fat: 12g
- Carbohydrates: 8g
- Fiber: 1g
- Serving Size: 4 servings
- Cooking Time: 20 minutes total

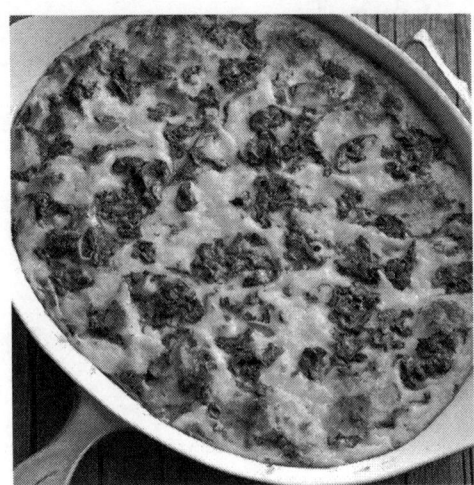

19. Rice Flour and Coconut Pancakes

Ingredients:
- 1 cup rice flour
- 1/2 cup coconut flour
- 2 teaspoons baking powder
- 1/4 teaspoon salt
- 1 cup coconut milk
- 2 eggs
- 2 tablespoons coconut oil, melted

Instructions:
1. In a bowl, mix rice flour, coconut flour, baking powder, and salt.
2. Add coconut milk, eggs, and melted coconut oil, whisking until the batter is smooth.
3. Heat a non-stick skillet or use the sauté function of the Instant Pot if available, and lightly grease it.
4. Pour batter to form pancakes and cook until bubbles form on the top, then flip to cook the other side until golden brown.
5. Serve warm.

Nutrition Info (Per Serving):
- Calories: 275
- Protein: 6g
- Fat: 16g
- Carbohydrates: 27g
- Fiber: 3g
- Serving Size: 4 servings
- Cooking Time: 20 minutes total (including preparation, not just pressure cooking)

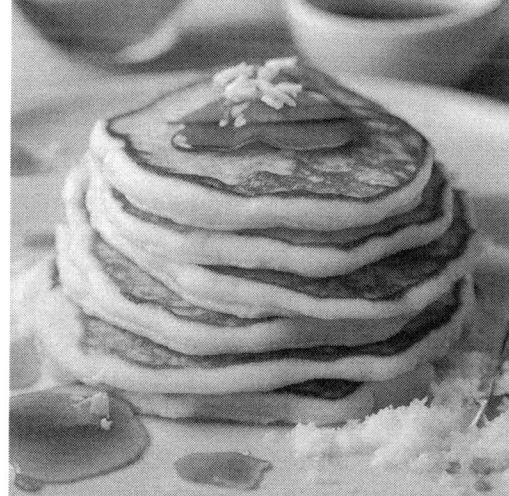

20. Herb-infused Breakfast Polenta

Ingredients:
- 1 cup polenta
- 4 cups water
- 1 teaspoon salt
- 1 tablespoon fresh rosemary, minced
- 1 tablespoon fresh thyme, minced
- 2 tablespoons olive oil

Instructions:
1. Add polenta, water, salt, rosemary, thyme, and olive oil to the Instant Pot.
2. Stir to combine all ingredients.
3. Close the lid, set the valve to sealing, and cook on Manual High Pressure for 7 minutes.
4. Allow the pressure to naturally release for 10 minutes, then quick release any remaining pressure.
5. Stir the polenta well before serving. It should be creamy and smooth.

Nutrition Info (Per Serving):
- Calories: 200
- Protein: 3g
- Fat: 7g
- Carbohydrates: 31g
- Fiber: 2g
- Serving Size: 4 servings
- Cooking Time: 17 minutes total

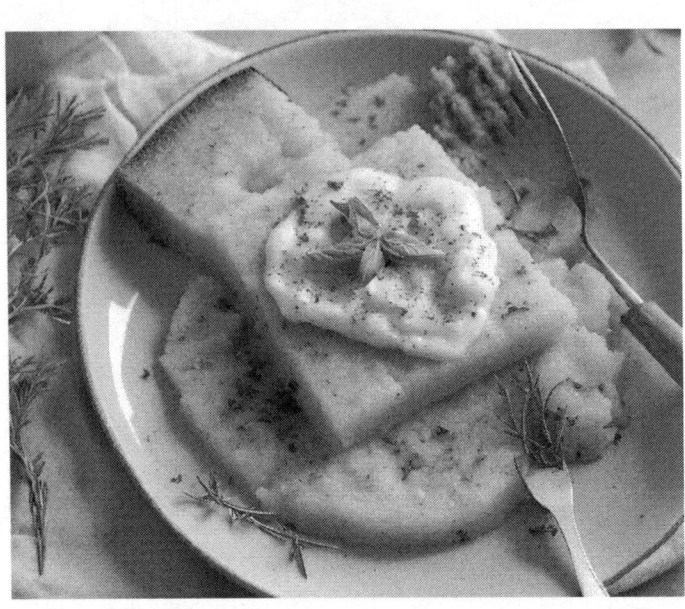

21. Pear and Cinnamon Breakfast Bars

Ingredients:
- 2 cups rolled oats
- 1 cup diced pears
- 1/2 cup almond flour
- 1/4 cup honey
- 1/2 teaspoon cinnamon
- 1/4 teaspoon salt
- 1/2 cup unsweetened applesauce
- 1/4 cup chopped walnuts (optional)

Instructions:
1. In a large bowl, combine rolled oats, almond flour, cinnamon, and salt.
2. Stir in diced pears, applesauce, honey, and walnuts until well mixed.
3. Transfer the mixture to a greased springform pan that fits inside your Instant Pot.
4. Pour 1 cup of water into the bottom of the Instant Pot and place the trivet inside.
5. Set the pan on the trivet, secure the lid, and set the valve to sealing.
6. Cook on Manual High Pressure for 25 minutes.
7. Let the pressure naturally release for 10 minutes, then quick release any remaining pressure.
8. Allow bars to cool in the pan before slicing and serving.

Nutrition Info (Per Serving):
- Calories: 180
- Protein: 4g
- Fat: 7g
- Carbohydrates: 28g
- Fiber: 4g
- Serving Size: 8 servings
- Cooking Time: 35 minutes total

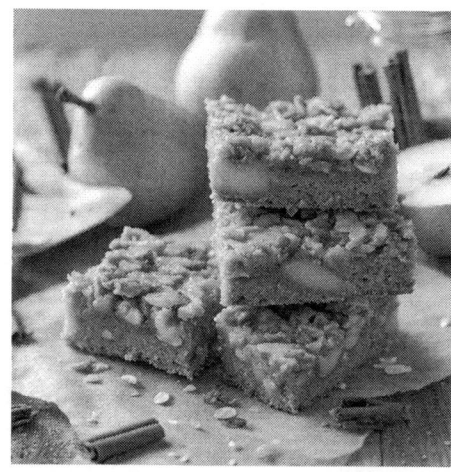

22. Carrot Cake Oatmeal

Ingredients:
- 1 cup steel-cut oats
- 3 cups water
- 1 cup grated carrots
- 1/2 teaspoon cinnamon
- 1/4 teaspoon nutmeg
- 2 tablespoons maple syrup (optional)
- 1/4 cup raisins
- 1/4 cup chopped walnuts

Instructions:
1. Add steel-cut oats, water, grated carrots, cinnamon, nutmeg, and maple syrup to the Instant Pot.
2. Stir to combine.
3. Close the lid, set the valve to sealing, and cook on Manual High Pressure for 10 minutes.
4. Allow the pressure to naturally release for 10 minutes, then quick release any remaining pressure.
5. Stir in raisins and chopped walnuts before serving.

Nutrition Info (Per Serving):
- Calories: 225
- Protein: 6g
- Fat: 5g
- Carbohydrates: 39g
- Fiber: 6g
- Serving Size: 4 servings
- Cooking Time: 20 minutes total

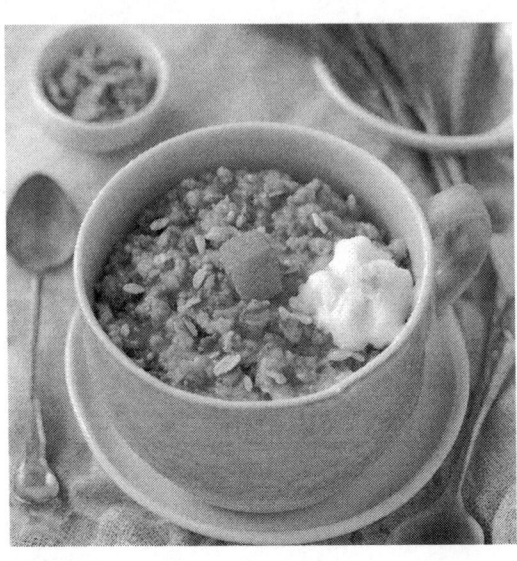

23. Savory Mushroom and Rice Breakfast Bowls

Ingredients:
- 1 cup brown rice, rinsed
- 2 cups vegetable broth
- 1 cup sliced mushrooms
- 1 onion, diced
- 1 garlic clove, minced
- 1 tablespoon olive oil
- Salt and pepper to taste
- 2 tablespoons chopped parsley (for garnish)

Instructions:
1. Set the Instant Pot to sauté mode and heat the olive oil.
2. Add the diced onion and garlic and sauté until translucent.
3. Add mushrooms and sauté until they begin to soften.
4. Stir in brown rice, vegetable broth, salt, and pepper.
5. Cancel sauté mode, secure the lid, set the valve to sealing, and cook on Manual High Pressure for 22 minutes.
6. Let the pressure naturally release for 10 minutes, then quick release any remaining pressure.
7. Stir the mixture, adjust seasoning if necessary, and garnish with chopped parsley before serving.

Nutrition Info (Per Serving):
- Calories: 215
- Protein: 5g
- Fat: 5g
- Carbohydrates: 37g
- Fiber: 3g
- Serving Size: 4 servings
- Cooking Time: 32 minutes total

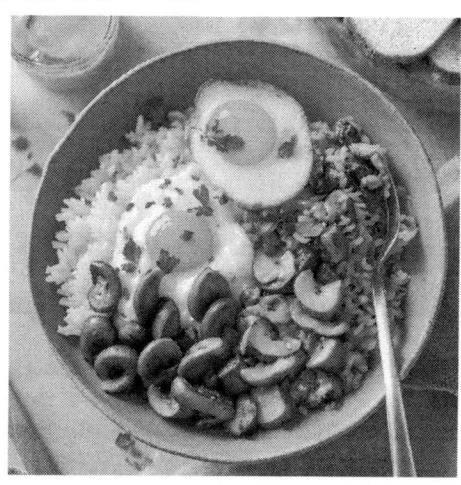

24. Peachy Keen Quinoa

Ingredients:
- 1 cup quinoa, rinsed
- 2 cups water
- 1 cup diced peaches (fresh or frozen)
- 1/2 teaspoon cinnamon
- 1 tablespoon honey
- 1/4 cup slivered almonds

Instructions:
1. Add quinoa, water, diced peaches, cinnamon, and honey to the Instant Pot.
2. Stir to mix all ingredients.
3. Secure the lid, set the valve to sealing, and cook on Manual High Pressure for 1 minute.
4. Allow the pressure to naturally release for 10 minutes, then quick release any remaining pressure.
5. Stir the quinoa well, sprinkle with slivered almonds, and serve.

Nutrition Info (Per Serving):
- Calories: 240
- Protein: 8g
- Fat: 5g
- Carbohydrates: 40g
- Fiber: 5g
- Serving Size: 4 servings
- Cooking Time: 11 minutes total

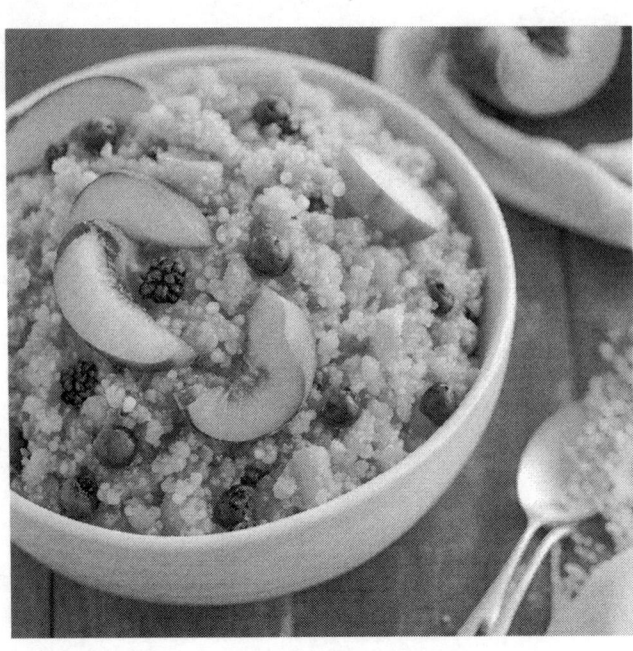

LUNCH

1. Lemon Herb Chicken and Rice
Ingredients:
- 2 tablespoons olive oil
- 4 boneless, skinless chicken breasts
- Juice of 1 lemon
- 1 teaspoon dried oregano
- 1 teaspoon dried basil
- 1 cup jasmine rice, rinsed
- 1 1/2 cups chicken broth
- Salt and pepper to taste
- Fresh parsley, chopped (for garnish)

Instructions:
1. Set the Instant Pot to sauté mode and heat the olive oil.
2. Season the chicken breasts with salt, pepper, oregano, and basil. Brown the chicken in the oil for about 2 minutes on each side.
3. Add the lemon juice, rinsed rice, and chicken broth to the pot.
4. Secure the lid, set the valve to sealing, and switch to the Manual High Pressure setting for 10 minutes.
5. Allow the Instant Pot to naturally release pressure for 10 minutes, then quick release any remaining pressure.
6. Serve the chicken and rice garnished with fresh parsley.

Nutrition Info (Per Serving):
- Calories: 410
- Protein: 30g
- Fat: 10g
- Carbohydrates: 45g
- Fiber: 1g
- Serving Size: 4 servings
- Cooking Time: 20 minutes total

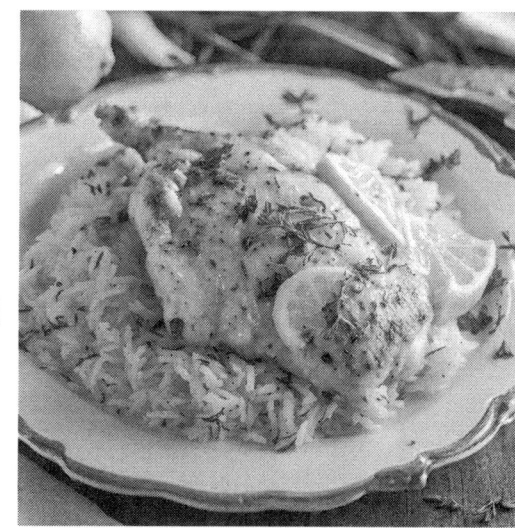

2. Butternut Squash Soup

Ingredients:
- 1 tablespoon olive oil
- 1 onion, diced
- 1 butternut squash, peeled and cubed (about 4 cups)
- 4 cups vegetable broth
- 1 teaspoon cinnamon
- 1/2 teaspoon nutmeg
- Salt and pepper to taste
- Coconut cream (optional, for serving)

Instructions:
1. Set the Instant Pot to sauté mode and heat the olive oil.
2. Add the onion and sauté until translucent.
3. Add the butternut squash, vegetable broth, cinnamon, nutmeg, salt, and pepper.
4. Secure the lid, set the valve to sealing, and cook on Manual High Pressure for 8 minutes.
5. Allow the pressure to naturally release for 10 minutes, then use the quick release for any remaining pressure.
6. Blend the soup using an immersion blender until smooth. Serve with a dollop of coconut cream if desired.

Nutrition Info (Per Serving):
- Calories: 150
- Protein: 2g
- Fat: 4g
- Carbohydrates: 28g
- Fiber: 5g
- Serving Size: 4 servings
- Cooking Time: 18 minutes total

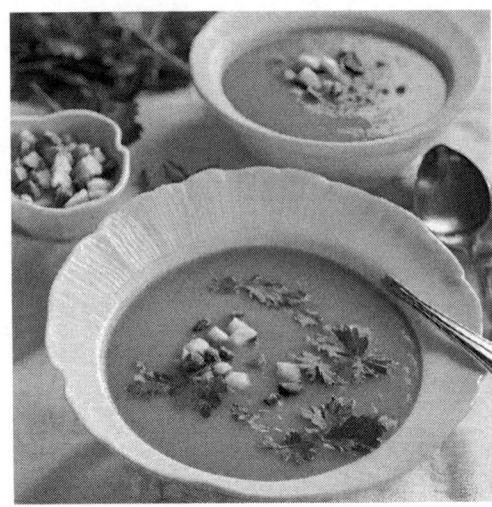

3. Beef and Sweet Potato Stew

Ingredients:
- 1 tablespoon olive oil
- 1 pound beef stew meat, cubed
- 2 sweet potatoes, peeled and cubed
- 1 onion, chopped
- 3 cups beef broth
- 1 teaspoon dried thyme
- 1 teaspoon dried rosemary
- Salt and pepper to taste

Instructions:
1. Set the Instant Pot to sauté mode and heat the olive oil.
2. Brown the beef stew meat on all sides.
3. Add the sweet potatoes, onion, beef broth, thyme, rosemary, salt, and pepper to the pot.
4. Secure the lid, set the valve to sealing, and cook on Manual High Pressure for 35 minutes.
5. Allow the pressure to naturally release for 15 minutes, then quick release any remaining pressure.
6. Serve the stew hot.

Nutrition Info (Per Serving):
- Calories: 350
- Protein: 28g
- Fat: 15g
- Carbohydrates: 22g
- Fiber: 3g
- Serving Size: 4 servings
- Cooking Time: 50 minutes total

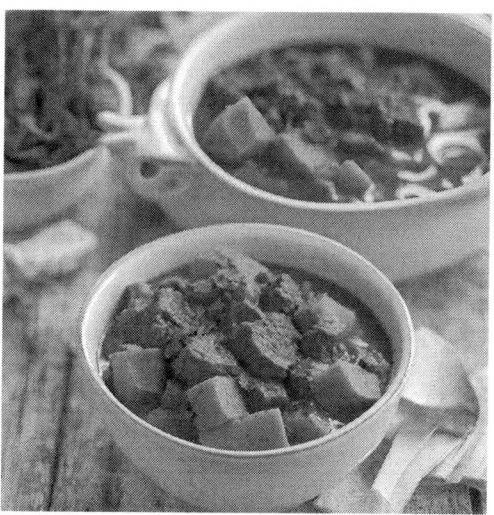

4. Quinoa Stuffed Bell Peppers

Ingredients:
- 4 large bell peppers, tops cut off and seeds removed
- 1 cup quinoa, rinsed
- 2 cups vegetable broth
- 1 onion, diced
- 1 zucchini, diced
- 1 teaspoon dried oregano
- 1/2 cup grated carrot
- Olive oil
- Salt and pepper to taste

Instructions:
1. In the Instant Pot, combine the quinoa and vegetable broth. Cook on Manual High Pressure for 1 minute.
2. Quick release the pressure, then set the Instant Pot to sauté mode.
3. Heat a little olive oil, then sauté the onion and zucchini until soft. Stir in the cooked quinoa, grated carrot, oregano, salt, and pepper.
4. Stuff the mixture into the bell peppers, place them in the Instant Pot on a trivet, and add 1 cup water to the pot.
5. Secure the lid, set the valve to sealing, and cook on Manual High Pressure for 8 minutes.
6. Quick release the pressure and serve the stuffed peppers.

Nutrition Info (Per Serving):
- Calories: 220
- Protein: 7g
- Fat: 5g
- Carbohydrates: 37g
- Fiber: 6g
- Serving Size: 4 servings
- Cooking Time: 20 minutes total

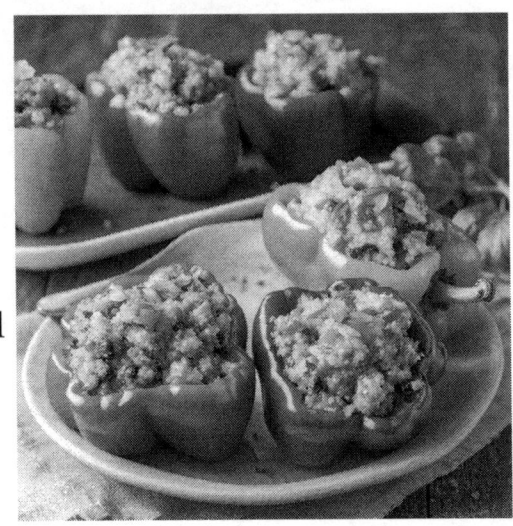

5. Chicken and Vegetable Broth

Ingredients:
- 2 pounds chicken bones or parts
- 1 onion, quartered
- 2 carrots, chopped
- 2 celery stalks, chopped
- 1 teaspoon salt
- 1/2 teaspoon pepper
- 6 cups water

Instructions:
1. Place all ingredients into the Instant Pot.
2. Fill with water until just covering the contents.
3. Secure the lid, set the valve to sealing, and cook on Manual High Pressure for 30 minutes.
4. Allow the pressure to naturally release for 20 minutes, then quick release any remaining pressure.
5. Strain the broth, discarding solids, and serve or use as a base for other dishes.

Nutrition Info (Per Serving):
- Calories: 50 (mostly from chicken)
- Protein: 6g
- Fat: 2g
- Carbohydrates: 3g
- Fiber: 1g
- Serving Size: 6 servings
- Cooking Time: 50 minutes total

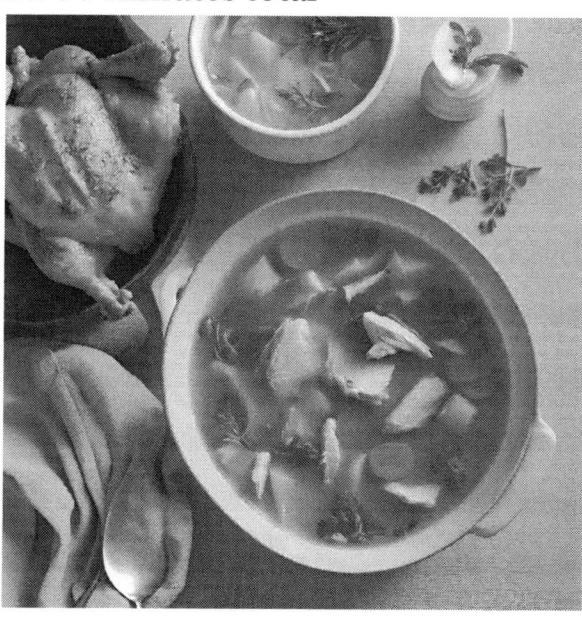

6. Ginger-Lime Cauliflower Rice

Ingredients:
- 1 head of cauliflower, riced
- 1 tablespoon olive oil
- 1 tablespoon fresh ginger, minced
- Juice and zest of 1 lime
- Salt and pepper to taste

Instructions:
1. Pulse cauliflower in a food processor until it resembles rice grains.
2. Set the Instant Pot to sauté mode and heat the olive oil.
3. Add the minced ginger and sauté for about 1 minute until fragrant.
4. Add the cauliflower rice, lime zest, and lime juice. Season with salt and pepper.
5. Sauté for about 3-5 minutes until the cauliflower is tender.
6. Cancel sauté mode, close the lid, and let sit for a few minutes to steam lightly before serving.

Nutrition Info (Per Serving):
- Calories: 70
- Protein: 2g
- Fat: 3.5g
- Carbohydrates: 9g
- Fiber: 3g
- Serving Size: 4 servings
- Cooking Time: 10 minutes total

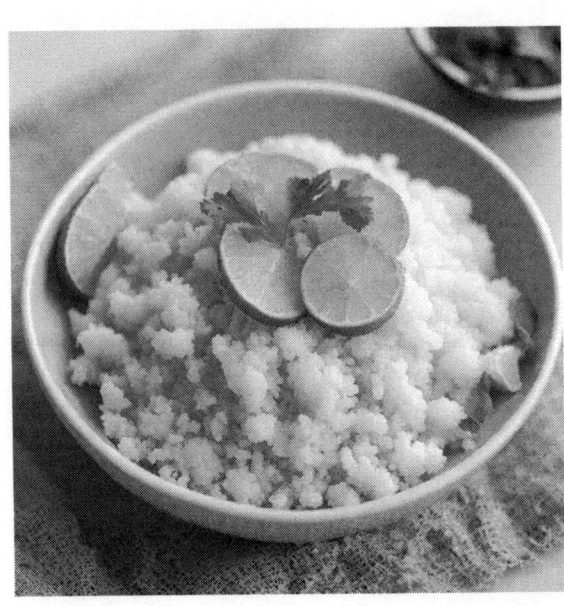

7. Parsley and Lemon Cod

Ingredients:
- 4 cod fillets
- Juice and zest of 1 lemon
- 1/4 cup chopped parsley
- 2 tablespoons olive oil
- Salt and pepper to taste

Instructions:
1. Pour 1 cup of water into the Instant Pot and insert the steam rack.
2. Place the cod fillets on the rack.
3. Drizzle with olive oil, and sprinkle lemon zest, chopped parsley, salt, and pepper over the cod.
4. Close the lid, set the valve to sealing, and steam using the "Steam" function for 4 minutes.
5. Quick release the pressure immediately after cooking.
6. Drizzle lemon juice over the fillets before serving.

Nutrition Info (Per Serving):
- Calories: 190
- Protein: 22g
- Fat: 10g
- Carbohydrates: 1g
- Fiber: 0g
- Serving Size: 4 servings
- Cooking Time: 9 minutes total

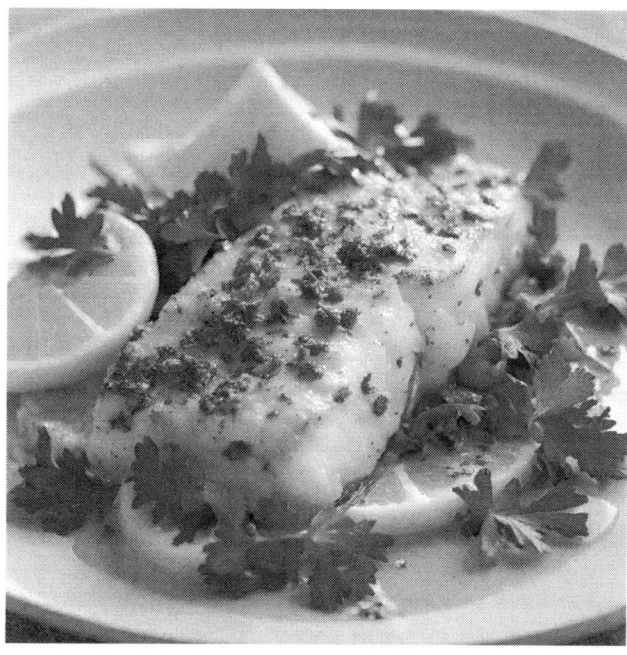

8. Carrot and Cumin Soup

Ingredients:
- 2 tablespoons olive oil
- 1 onion, chopped
- 4 cups chopped carrots
- 1 teaspoon ground cumin
- 4 cups vegetable broth
- Salt and pepper to taste

Instructions:
1. Set the Instant Pot to sauté mode and heat the olive oil.
2. Add the onion and sauté until translucent.
3. Add the carrots and cumin, stirring for a few minutes until fragrant.
4. Pour in the vegetable broth and season with salt and pepper.
5. Close the lid, set the valve to sealing, and cook on Manual High Pressure for 15 minutes.
6. Quick release the pressure, then puree the soup using an immersion blender until smooth.
7. Adjust seasoning if necessary and serve hot.

Nutrition Info (Per Serving):
- Calories: 130
- Protein: 2g
- Fat: 7g
- Carbohydrates: 15g
- Fiber: 4g
- Serving Size: 4 servings
- Cooking Time: 25 minutes total

9. Turkey and Pumpkin Chili

Ingredients:
- 1 pound ground turkey
- 1 onion, diced
- 2 cups pumpkin puree
- 1 can (15 oz) diced tomatoes
- 1 cup chicken broth
- 1 tablespoon chili powder
- 1 teaspoon cumin
- 1/2 teaspoon cinnamon
- Salt and pepper to taste

Instructions:
1. Set the Instant Pot to sauté mode and brown the ground turkey with the diced onion.
2. Add pumpkin puree, diced tomatoes, chicken broth, chili powder, cumin, and cinnamon.
3. Stir to combine all ingredients and season with salt and pepper.
4. Close the lid, set the valve to sealing, and cook on Manual High Pressure for 20 minutes.
5. Allow the pressure to naturally release for 10 minutes, then quick release any remaining pressure.
6. Stir well before serving.

Nutrition Info (Per Serving):
- Calories: 250
- Protein: 23g
- Fat: 8g
- Carbohydrates: 23g
- Fiber: 5g
- Serving Size: 4 servings
- Cooking Time: 40 minutes total

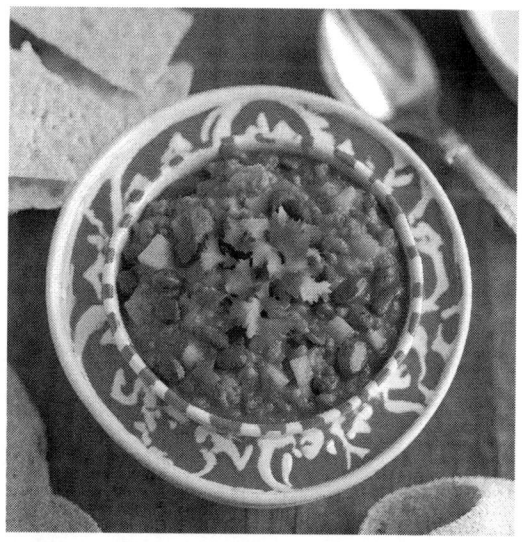

10. Zucchini and Basil Risotto

Ingredients:
- 1 tablespoon olive oil
- 1 onion, finely chopped
- 1 cup Arborio rice
- 3 cups vegetable broth
- 1 zucchini, diced
- 1/2 cup fresh basil, chopped
- 1/4 cup grated Parmesan cheese (optional)
- Salt and pepper to taste

Instructions:
1. Set the Instant Pot to sauté mode and heat the olive oil.
2. Add the onion and sauté until translucent.
3. Add the Arborio rice, stirring for a minute to coat the grains in oil.
4. Pour in the vegetable broth and add the diced zucchini.
5. Close the lid, set the valve to sealing, and cook on the "Risotto" or Manual High Pressure setting for 6 minutes.
6. Quick release the pressure, then stir in the chopped basil and Parmesan cheese.
7. Season with salt and pepper to taste and serve immediately.

Nutrition Info (Per Serving):
- Calories: 300
- Protein: 7g
- Fat: 8g
- Carbohydrates: 50g
- Fiber: 2g
- Serving Size: 4 servings
- Cooking Time: 16 minutes total

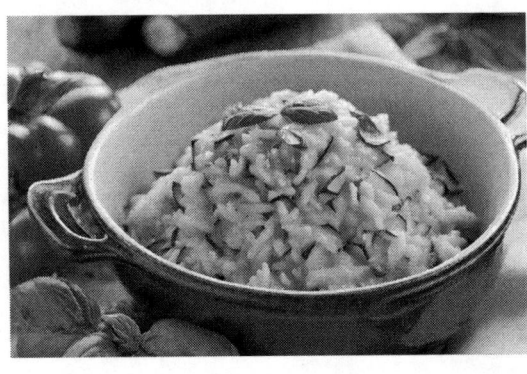

11. Instant Pot Spaghetti Squash and Meat Sauce

Ingredients:
- 1 medium spaghetti squash, halved and seeds removed
- 1 pound ground beef
- 1 onion, chopped
- 2 cloves garlic, minced
- 1 can (28 oz) crushed tomatoes
- 1 teaspoon dried basil
- 1 teaspoon dried oregano
- Salt and pepper to taste
- 1 cup water

Instructions:
1. Pour the water into the Instant Pot and place the trivet inside. Set the squash halves on the trivet, cut side up.
2. Set the Instant Pot to sauté mode and brown the ground beef with onion and garlic in a separate skillet or use another pot if your model has a sauté function.
3. Add crushed tomatoes, basil, oregano, salt, and pepper to the beef, stirring to combine.
4. Secure the lid on the Instant Pot, ensuring the valve is set to sealing, and cook on Manual High Pressure for 15 minutes.
5. Allow the pressure to naturally release for 10 minutes, then quick release any remaining pressure.
6. Use a fork to shred the inside of the squash into spaghetti-like strands.
7. Serve the spaghetti squash topped with the meat sauce.

Nutrition Info (Per Serving):
- Calories: 320
- Protein: 23g
- Fat: 15g
- Carbohydrates: 22g
- Fiber: 6g
- Serving Size: 4 servings
- Cooking Time: 35 minutes total

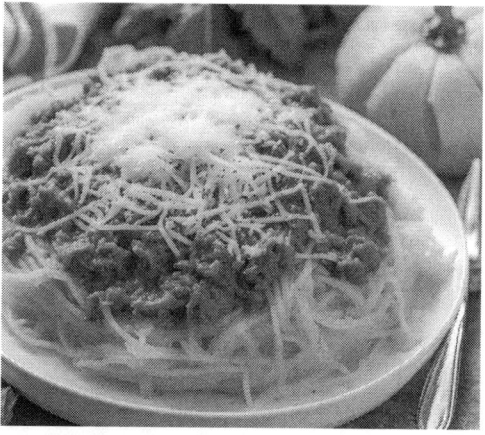

12. Turkey Meatball Soup

Ingredients:
- 1 pound ground turkey
- 1/4 cup breadcrumbs
- 1 egg
- 1 teaspoon dried oregano
- 1 teaspoon dried basil
- 4 cups chicken broth
- 1 cup chopped carrots
- 1 cup chopped celery
- Salt and pepper to taste

Instructions:
1. In a bowl, combine ground turkey, breadcrumbs, egg, oregano, basil, salt, and pepper. Mix well and form into small meatballs.
2. Pour the chicken broth into the Instant Pot and add the meatballs along with the chopped carrots and celery.
3. Secure the lid, set the valve to sealing, and cook on Manual High Pressure for 7 minutes.
4. Quick release the pressure once cooking is complete.
5. Adjust seasoning as needed and serve hot.

Nutrition Info (Per Serving):
- Calories: 270
- Protein: 28g
- Fat: 12g
- Carbohydrates: 10g
- Fiber: 2g
- Serving Size: 4 servings
- Cooking Time: 17 minutes total

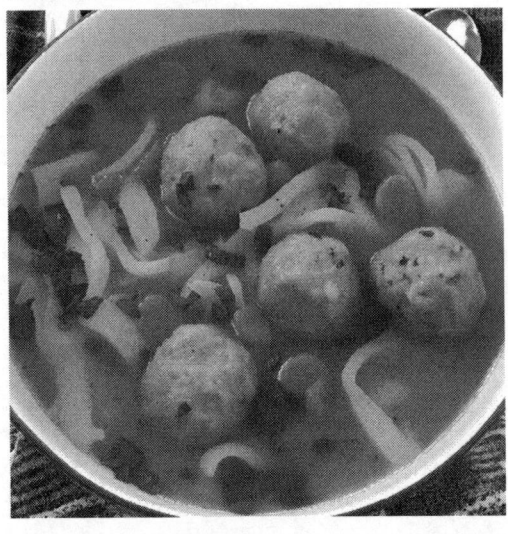

13. Butternut Squash and Ginger Porridge

Ingredients:
- 1 cup steel-cut oats
- 3 cups water
- 2 cups peeled and cubed butternut squash
- 1 tablespoon grated ginger
- 1 teaspoon cinnamon
- 1/4 cup maple syrup (optional)

Instructions:
1. Add steel-cut oats, water, butternut squash, ginger, and cinnamon to the Instant Pot.
2. Stir to combine all ingredients.
3. Close the lid, set the valve to sealing, and cook on Manual High Pressure for 10 minutes.
4. Allow the pressure to naturally release for 10 minutes, then quick release any remaining pressure.
5. Stir in maple syrup if using before serving.

Nutrition Info (Per Serving):
- Calories: 210
- Protein: 6g
- Fat: 2g
- Carbohydrates: 43g
- Fiber: 6g
- Serving Size: 4 servings
- Cooking Time: 20 minutes total

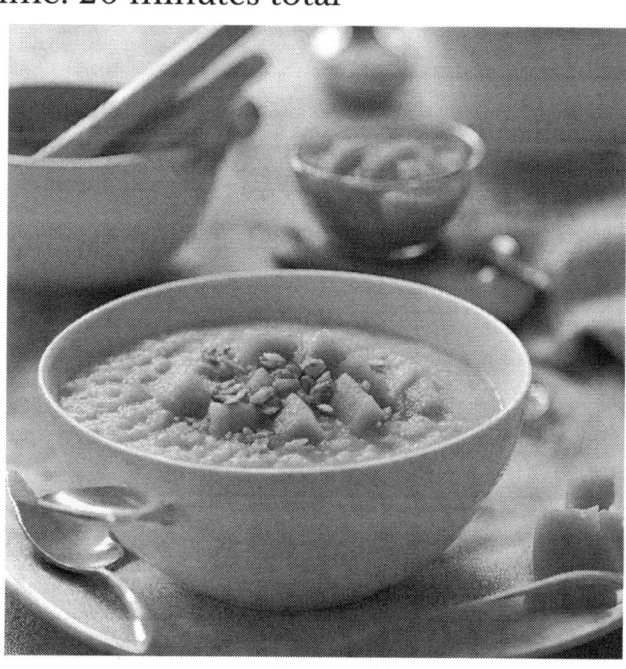

14. Sweet Potato and Chicken Curry
Ingredients:
- 2 tablespoons olive oil
- 1 onion, chopped
- 2 cloves garlic, minced
- 1 pound boneless skinless chicken breasts, cut into cubes
- 2 large sweet potatoes, peeled and cubed
- 1 can (14 oz) coconut milk
- 2 tablespoons curry powder
- 1 teaspoon turmeric
- Salt and pepper to taste
- 1 cup water

Instructions:
1. Set the Instant Pot to sauté mode and heat the olive oil.
2. Add onion and garlic, and sauté until soft.
3. Add chicken and brown slightly.
4. Stir in sweet potatoes, coconut milk, curry powder, turmeric, salt, pepper, and water.
5. Secure the lid, set the valve to sealing, and cook on Manual High Pressure for 8 minutes.
6. Quick release the pressure carefully after cooking.
7. Stir the curry well and adjust seasoning if necessary before serving.

Nutrition Info (Per Serving):
- Calories: 390
- Protein: 28g
- Fat: 20g
- Carbohydrates: 28g
- Fiber: 5g
- Serving Size: 4 servings
- Cooking Time: 18 minutes total

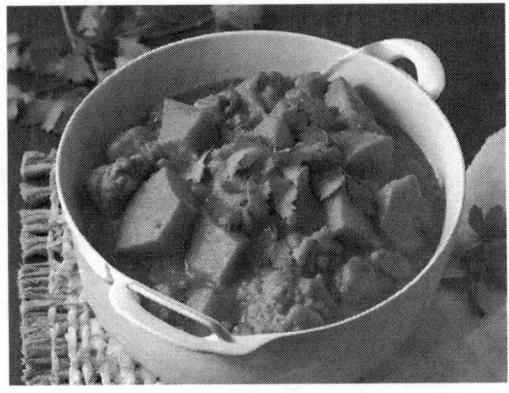

15. Lemon Garlic Shrimp and Asparagus

Ingredients:
- 1 pound large shrimp, peeled and deveined
- 1 bunch asparagus, trimmed and cut into 1-inch pieces
- 4 cloves garlic, minced
- Juice and zest of 1 lemon
- 2 tablespoons olive oil
- Salt and pepper to taste

Instructions:
1. Set the Instant Pot to sauté mode and heat the olive oil.
2. Add the garlic and sauté for 1 minute until fragrant.
3. Add the shrimp and asparagus, lemon zest, and lemon juice. Season with salt and pepper.
4. Sauté for 3-4 minutes until the shrimp start to turn pink.
5. Close the lid, set the valve to sealing, and cook on Manual High Pressure for 2 minutes.
6. Quick release the pressure immediately after cooking.
7. Serve the shrimp and asparagus hot, garnished with additional lemon slices if desired.

Nutrition Info (Per Serving):
- Calories: 180
- Protein: 24g
- Fat: 8g
- Carbohydrates: 5g
- Fiber: 2g
- Serving Size: 4 servings
- Cooking Time: 10 minutes total

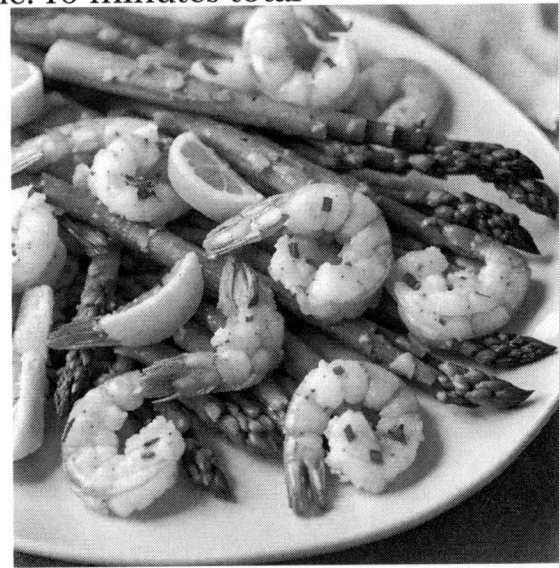

16. Minty Pea Soup

Ingredients:
- 2 tablespoons olive oil
- 1 onion, chopped
- 4 cups frozen peas
- 4 cups vegetable broth
- 1/2 cup fresh mint leaves
- Salt and pepper to taste

Instructions:
1. Set the Instant Pot to sauté mode and heat the olive oil.
2. Add the onion and sauté until soft and translucent.
3. Add the peas, vegetable broth, and mint leaves. Season with salt and pepper.
4. Close the lid, set the valve to sealing, and cook on Manual High Pressure for 5 minutes.
5. Quick release the pressure, then puree the soup using an immersion blender until smooth.
6. Adjust seasoning if necessary and serve hot.

Nutrition Info (Per Serving):
- Calories: 160
- Protein: 8g
- Fat: 5g
- Carbohydrates: 22g
- Fiber: 8g
- Serving Size: 4 servings
- Cooking Time: 15 minutes total

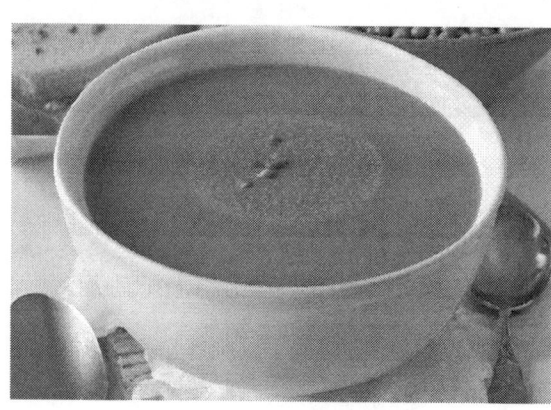

17. Beef Stroganoff with Coconut Cream

Ingredients:
- 1 pound beef stew meat, cut into 1-inch cubes
- 1 onion, sliced
- 2 cloves garlic, minced
- 1 cup beef broth
- 1 tablespoon paprika
- 1 cup coconut cream
- 1 tablespoon Dijon mustard
- 1 cup sliced mushrooms
- Salt and pepper to taste
- 2 tablespoons fresh parsley, chopped (for garnish)

Instructions:
1. Set the Instant Pot to sauté mode and brown the beef on all sides.
2. Add the onion, garlic, and mushrooms, and sauté for a few minutes until soft.
3. Add the beef broth, paprika, and season with salt and pepper.
4. Close the lid, set the valve to sealing, and cook on Manual High Pressure for 15 minutes.
5. Quick release the pressure, stir in the coconut cream and Dijon mustard.
6. Set the pot to sauté mode again and let it simmer for a few minutes until the sauce thickens.
7. Serve garnished with fresh parsley.

Nutrition Info (Per Serving):
- Calories: 350
- Protein: 25g
- Fat: 25g
- Carbohydrates: 8g
- Fiber: 1g
- Serving Size: 4 servings
- Cooking Time: 30 minutes total

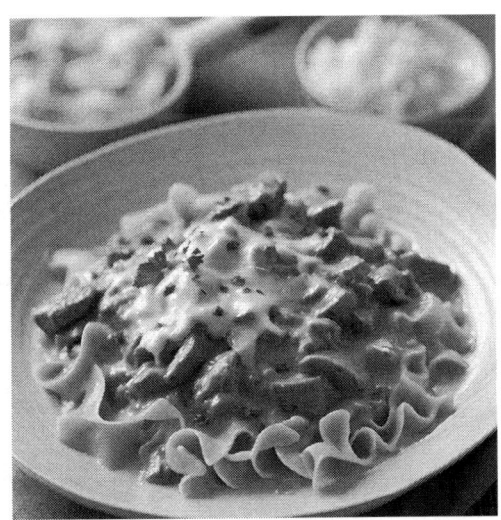

18. Herbed Chicken Salad

Ingredients:
- 2 pounds boneless skinless chicken breasts
- 1/2 cup chicken broth
- Juice of 1 lemon
- 1/4 cup chopped fresh herbs (parsley, dill, chives)
- 1/2 cup Greek yogurt
- 1/4 cup chopped celery
- Salt and pepper to taste

Instructions:
1. Place chicken breasts, chicken broth, and lemon juice in the Instant Pot.
2. Close the lid, set the valve to sealing, and cook on Manual High Pressure for 10 minutes.
3. Allow natural pressure release for 10 minutes, then quick release any remaining pressure.
4. Remove the chicken, let it cool, and then shred it with forks.
5. In a bowl, mix shredded chicken with Greek yogurt, celery, fresh herbs, salt, and pepper.
6. Serve chilled, garnished with extra herbs if desired.

Nutrition Info (Per Serving):
- Calories: 245
- Protein: 38g
- Fat: 7g
- Carbohydrates: 5g
- Fiber: 1g
- Serving Size: 6 servings
- Cooking Time: 20 minutes total

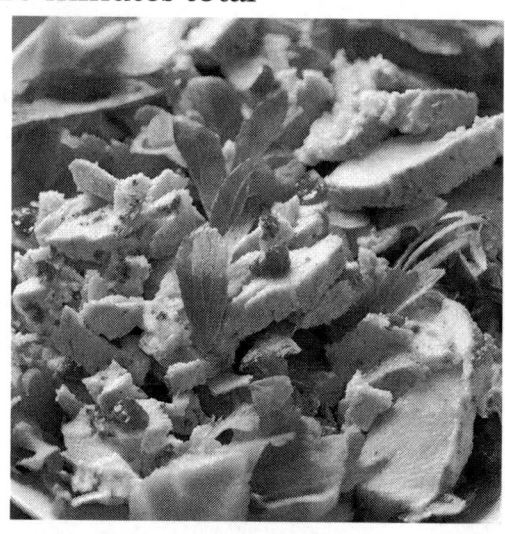

19. Lentil and Carrot Stew

Ingredients:
- 1 tablespoon olive oil
- 1 onion, chopped
- 2 cloves garlic, minced
- 2 carrots, diced
- 1 cup dried lentils, rinsed
- 4 cups vegetable broth
- 1 teaspoon ground cumin
- 1/2 teaspoon ground coriander
- Salt and pepper to taste
- 2 tablespoons fresh parsley, chopped (for garnish)

Instructions:
1. Set the Instant Pot to sauté mode and heat the olive oil.
2. Add the onion and garlic, sautéing until translucent.
3. Add the carrots and sauté for a few more minutes.
4. Stir in the lentils, vegetable broth, cumin, and coriander. Season with salt and pepper.
5. Close the lid, set the valve to sealing, and cook on Manual High Pressure for 15 minutes.
6. Allow natural pressure release for 10 minutes, then quick release any remaining pressure.
7. Stir well, adjust seasoning if necessary, and serve garnished with fresh parsley.

Nutrition Info (Per Serving):
- Calories: 220
- Protein: 12g
- Fat: 3g
- Carbohydrates: 35g
- Fiber: 15g
- Serving Size: 4 servings
- Cooking Time: 30 minutes total

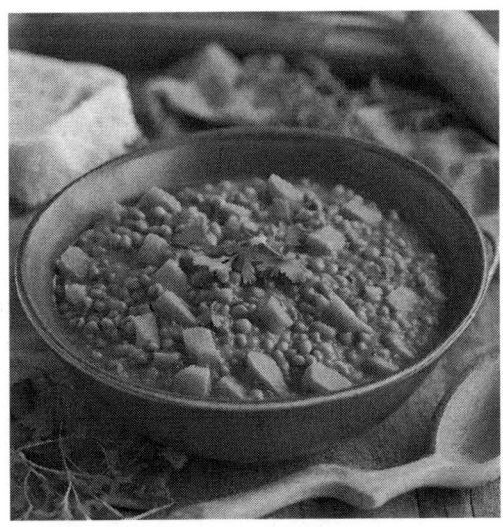

20. Balsamic Glazed Pork Tenderloin

Ingredients:
- 1 pork tenderloin (about 1 pound)
- Salt and pepper to taste
- 1 tablespoon olive oil
- 1/4 cup balsamic vinegar
- 2 tablespoons honey
- 1 clove garlic, minced
- 1 teaspoon dried thyme

Instructions:
1. Season the pork tenderloin with salt and pepper.
2. Set the Instant Pot to sauté mode and heat the olive oil. Brown the pork on all sides.
3. Mix balsamic vinegar, honey, garlic, and thyme together in a bowl.
4. Pour the balsamic mixture over the pork in the pot.
5. Close the lid, set the valve to sealing, and cook on Manual High Pressure for 10 minutes.
6. Allow natural pressure release for 10 minutes, then quick release any remaining pressure.
7. Remove the pork, slice, and drizzle with the thickened balsamic glaze from the pot before serving.

Nutrition Info (Per Serving):
- Calories: 265
- Protein: 24g
- Fat: 12g
- Carbohydrates: 15g
- Fiber: 0g
- Serving Size: 4 servings
- Cooking Time: 20 minutes total

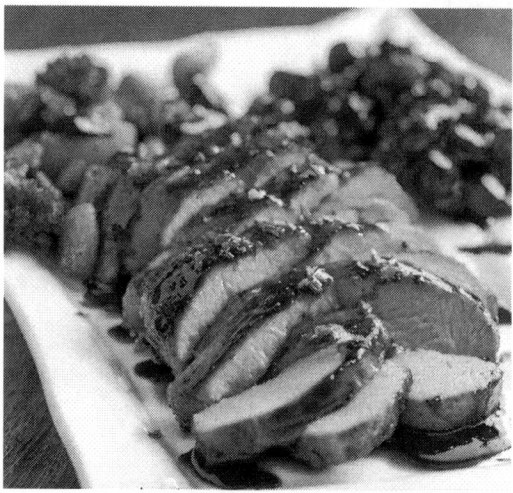

21. Instant Pot Kale and Potato Soup

Ingredients:
- 1 tablespoon olive oil
- 1 onion, chopped
- 2 cloves garlic, minced
- 4 cups chopped kale
- 2 large potatoes, peeled and diced
- 4 cups vegetable broth
- Salt and pepper to taste

Instructions:
1. Set the Instant Pot to sauté mode and heat the olive oil.
2. Add the onion and garlic, and sauté until softened.
3. Add the kale and potatoes, stirring to combine.
4. Pour in the vegetable broth, and season with salt and pepper.
5. Close the lid, set the valve to sealing, and cook on Manual High Pressure for 10 minutes.
6. Quick release the pressure, then puree the soup if desired for a smoother texture or serve as is for a chunkier soup.

Nutrition Info (Per Serving):
- Calories: 180
- Protein: 6g
- Fat: 3g
- Carbohydrates: 35g
- Fiber: 6g
- Serving Size: 4 servings
- Cooking Time: 20 minutes total

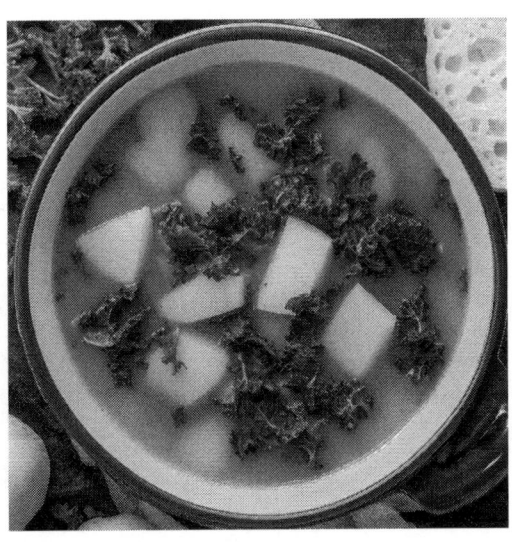

22. Herb-Infused Turkey Breast

Ingredients:
- 1 turkey breast (about 3 pounds)
- 2 tablespoons olive oil
- 1 tablespoon chopped fresh rosemary
- 1 tablespoon chopped fresh thyme
- 1 clove garlic, minced
- Salt and pepper to taste
- 1 cup chicken broth

Instructions:
1. Rub the turkey breast with olive oil, minced garlic, rosemary, thyme, salt, and pepper.
2. Pour chicken broth into the Instant Pot and place the trivet inside.
3. Set the turkey breast on the trivet.
4. Close the lid, set the valve to sealing, and cook on Manual High Pressure for 25 minutes.
5. Allow natural pressure release for 20 minutes, then quick release any remaining pressure.
6. Remove the turkey, let it rest for a few minutes, then slice and serve.

Nutrition Info (Per Serving):
- Calories: 320
- Protein: 45g
- Fat: 14g
- Carbohydrates: 2g
- Fiber: 0g
- Serving Size: 6 servings
- Cooking Time: 45 minutes total

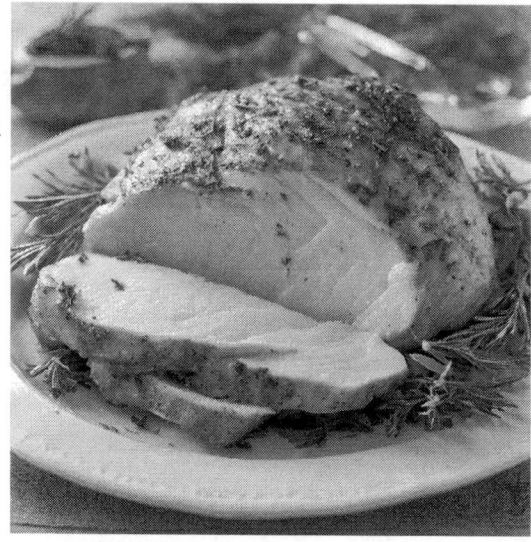

23. Quinoa Vegetable Pilaf

Ingredients:
- 1 tablespoon olive oil
- 1 onion, diced
- 1 carrot, diced
- 1 red bell pepper, diced
- 1 cup quinoa, rinsed
- 2 cups vegetable broth
- 1 teaspoon dried thyme
- Salt and pepper to taste
- 1/4 cup chopped fresh parsley

Instructions:
1. Set the Instant Pot to sauté mode and heat the olive oil.
2. Add the onion, carrot, and bell pepper, sautéing until softened.
3. Stir in the quinoa, vegetable broth, thyme, salt, and pepper.
4. Close the lid, set the valve to sealing, and cook on Manual High Pressure for 1 minute.
5. Allow natural pressure release for 10 minutes, then quick release any remaining pressure.
6. Stir in the fresh parsley before serving.

Nutrition Info (Per Serving):
- Calories: 220
- Protein: 8g
- Fat: 5g
- Carbohydrates: 36g
- Fiber: 5g
- Serving Size: 4 servings
- Cooking Time: 16 minutes total

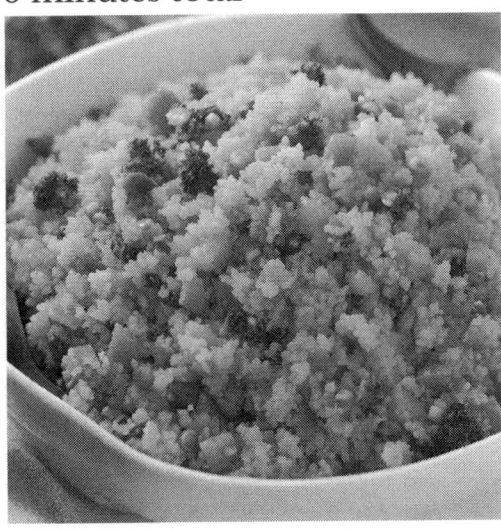

24. Moroccan-Inspired Chicken Stew
Ingredients:
- 2 tablespoons olive oil
- 1 onion, chopped
- 2 cloves garlic, minced
- 1 pound chicken thighs, cut into pieces
- 2 teaspoons ground cumin
- 1 teaspoon ground cinnamon
- 1/2 teaspoon ground ginger
- 1 can (15 oz) diced tomatoes
- 1 can (15 oz) chickpeas, drained and rinsed
- 1/2 cup dried apricots, chopped
- 2 cups chicken broth
- Salt and pepper to taste
- Fresh cilantro for garnish

Instructions:
1. Set the Instant Pot to sauté mode and heat the olive oil.
2. Add the onion and garlic, sautéing until translucent.
3. Add the chicken and brown slightly.
4. Stir in cumin, cinnamon, and ginger, cooking for another minute until fragrant.
5. Add tomatoes, chickpeas, apricots, and chicken broth. Season with salt and pepper.
6. Close the lid, set the valve to sealing, and cook on Manual High Pressure for 15 minutes.
7. Allow natural pressure release for 10 minutes, then quick release any remaining pressure.
8. Serve the stew garnished with fresh cilantro.

Nutrition Info (Per Serving):
- Calories: 350
- Protein: 28g
- Fat: 15g
- Carbohydrates: 27g
- Fiber: 6g
- Serving Size: 4 servings
- Cooking Time: 30 minutes total

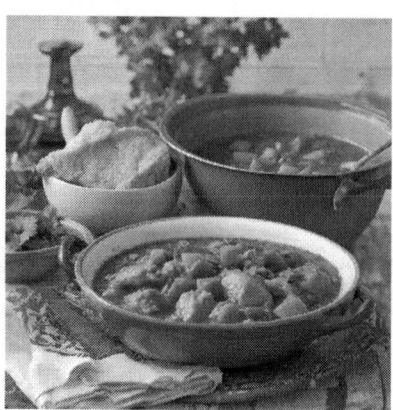

25. Beetroot and Carrot Salad

Ingredients:
- 3 beetroots, peeled and grated
- 3 carrots, peeled and grated
- 1/4 cup olive oil
- Juice of 1 lemon
- 1 teaspoon Dijon mustard
- Salt and pepper to taste
- 1/4 cup chopped walnuts (optional)

Instructions:
1. Mix the grated beetroots and carrots in a salad bowl.
2. In a small bowl, whisk together olive oil, lemon juice, Dijon mustard, salt, and pepper to create the dressing.
3. Pour the dressing over the beetroot and carrot mixture and toss well.
4. Garnish with chopped walnuts if using and serve chilled.

Nutrition Info (Per Serving):
- Calories: 180
- Protein: 2g
- Fat: 14g
- Carbohydrates: 13g
- Fiber: 4g
- Serving Size: 4 servings
- Cooking Time: 5 minutes total (no cooking, just preparation)

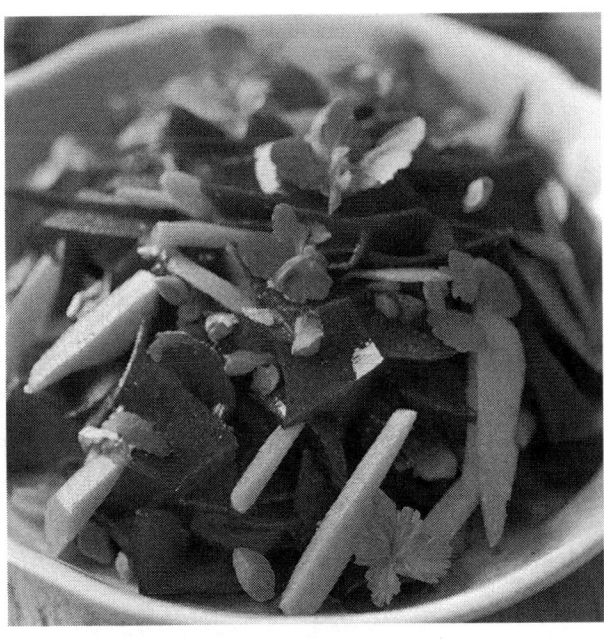

26. Instant Pot Lemon Pepper Cod

Ingredients:
- 4 cod fillets
- Juice and zest of 1 lemon
- 1 teaspoon black pepper
- 1/2 cup water
- Salt to taste
- Parsley for garnish

Instructions:
1. Season the cod fillets with lemon zest, black pepper, and salt.
2. Pour water into the Instant Pot and place the trivet inside.
3. Place the seasoned cod on the trivet.
4. Close the lid, set the valve to sealing, and cook on Manual High Pressure for 2 minutes.
5. Quick release the pressure immediately after cooking.
6. Drizzle lemon juice over the cooked cod and garnish with parsley before serving.

Nutrition Info (Per Serving):
- Calories: 120
- Protein: 23g
- Fat: 1g
- Carbohydrates: 1g
- Fiber: 0g
- Serving Size: 4 servings
- Cooking Time: 7 minutes total

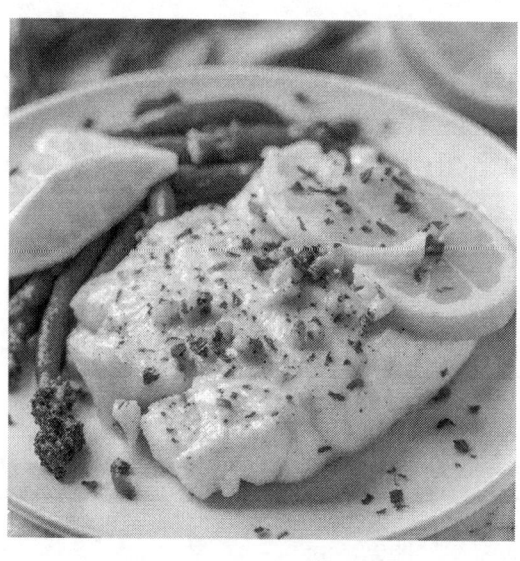

27. Saffron Rice with Vegetables

Ingredients:
- 1 cup basmati rice, rinsed
- 1 3/4 cups water
- A pinch of saffron threads, soaked in 2 tablespoons hot water
- 1 tablespoon olive oil
- 1/2 cup diced carrots
- 1/2 cup peas
- Salt to taste

Instructions:
1. Set the Instant Pot to sauté mode and heat the olive oil.
2. Add the carrots and sauté for a few minutes.
3. Add the rinsed rice, saffron water, and additional water. Stir in the peas and season with salt.
4. Close the lid, set the valve to sealing, and cook on Manual High Pressure for 4 minutes.
5. Allow natural pressure release for 10 minutes, then quick release any remaining pressure.
6. Fluff the rice gently and serve.

Nutrition Info (Per Serving):
- Calories: 220
- Protein: 4g
- Fat: 4g
- Carbohydrates: 40g
- Fiber: 2g
- Serving Size: 4 servings
- Cooking Time: 19 minutes total

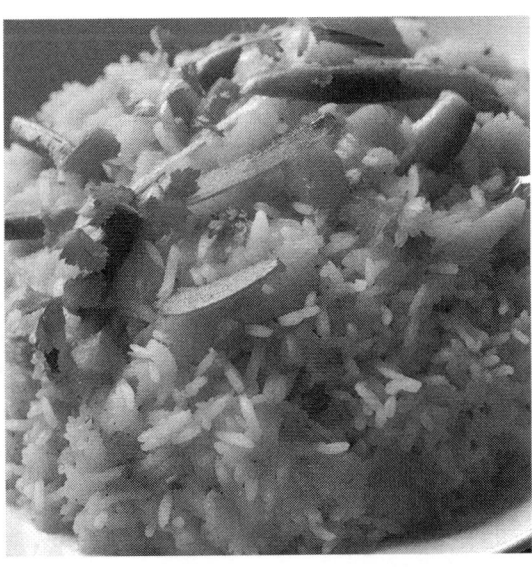

DINNER

1. Fennel and Orange Salad with Grilled Chicken
Ingredients:
- 2 boneless, skinless chicken breasts
- 1 fennel bulb, thinly sliced
- 2 oranges, peeled and segments cut out
- 1/4 cup olive oil, plus extra for grilling
- 2 tablespoons white wine vinegar
- 1 teaspoon honey (optional, depending on histamine tolerance)
- Salt and pepper to taste
- Mixed greens for serving

Instructions:
1. Season the chicken breasts with salt and pepper and drizzle with olive oil.
2. Set the Instant Pot to sauté mode and place the chicken in the pot once it's hot. Grill each side for about 3-4 minutes until golden and fully cooked.
3. Remove the chicken and let it rest while you assemble the salad.
4. In a large bowl, combine the sliced fennel, orange segments, and mixed greens.
5. In a small bowl, whisk together 1/4 cup olive oil, white wine vinegar, honey, salt, and pepper to create the dressing.
6. Slice the grilled chicken and add it to the salad.
7. Drizzle the dressing over the salad, toss gently to coat, and serve.

Nutrition Info (Per Serving):
Calories: 350 Protein: 26g Fat: 23g Carbohydrates: 15g Fiber: 5g
- Serving Size: 4 servings
- Cooking Time: 10 minutes (plus assembly time)

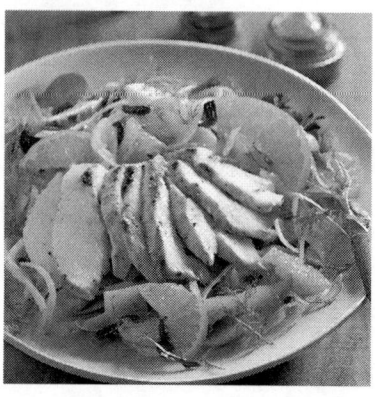

2. Instant Pot Lemon Thyme Chicken

Instructions :
1. Sear the chicken on each side for about 2 minutes until golden.
2. Pour in the lemon juice and chicken broth, scraping up any brown bits from the bottom of the pot.
3. Close the lid, set the valve to sealing, and switch to Manual High Pressure for 7 minutes.
4. After the cooking time is over, allow the Instant Pot to naturally release pressure for 10 minutes, then manually release any remaining steam.
5. Remove the chicken breasts, and if desired, you can thicken the sauce left in the pot by setting the Instant Pot to sauté mode and simmering until reduced to your liking.
6. Serve the chicken drizzled with the thickened sauce.

Nutrition Info (Per Serving):
- Calories: 240
- Protein: 29g
- Fat: 11g
- Carbohydrates: 3g
- Fiber: 0g
- Serving Size: 4 servings
- Cooking Time: 20 minutes total (includes sautéing, pressure cooking, and natural release)

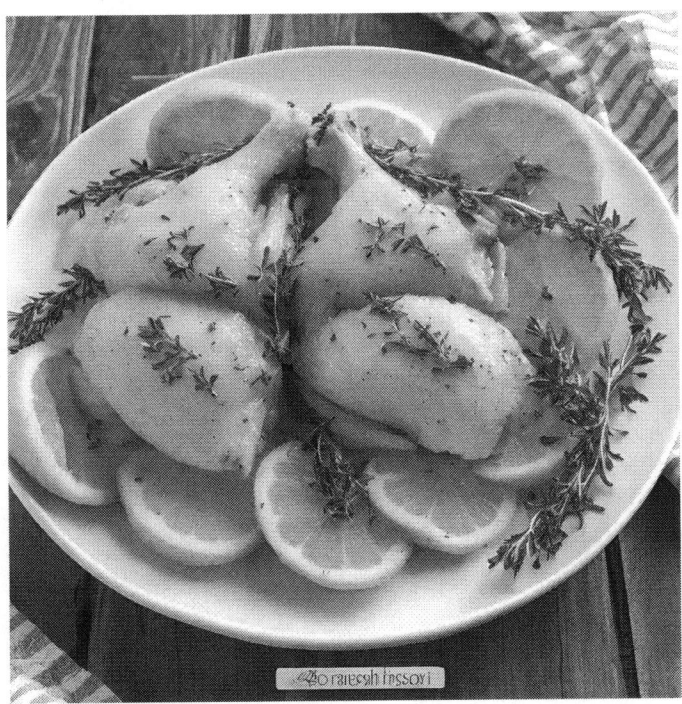

3. Garlic-Infused Mashed Potatoes

Ingredients:
- 2 pounds Yukon Gold potatoes, peeled and cubed
- 4 cloves garlic, minced
- 1 cup water
- 1/2 cup milk (or dairy-free alternative)
- 1/4 cup butter (or vegan butter)
- Salt and pepper to taste
- Fresh chives, chopped for garnish

Instructions:
1. Place the cubed potatoes and minced garlic in the Instant Pot.
2. Add 1 cup of water and sprinkle with salt.
3. Secure the lid, set the valve to sealing, and cook on Manual High Pressure for 8 minutes.
4. Once the cooking time is complete, quick release the pressure and drain the potatoes, reserving some of the cooking liquid.
5. Add the milk and butter to the potatoes. Mash the potatoes, adding the reserved cooking liquid as needed to reach your desired consistency.
6. Season with salt and pepper to taste, and mix thoroughly.
7. Garnish with chopped chives and serve hot.

Nutrition Info (Per Serving):
- Calories: 250
- Protein: 4g
- Fat: 11g
- Carbohydrates: 34g
- Fiber: 3g
- Serving Size: 6 servings
- Cooking Time: 18 minutes total (includes pressure build-up, cooking, and release)

4. Bok Choy and Shiitake Mushroom Stir-Fry

Ingredients:
- 2 tablespoons olive oil
- 4 cups bok choy, chopped
- 2 cups shiitake mushrooms, sliced
- 2 cloves garlic, minced
- 2 tablespoons soy sauce (or a low histamine alternative like coconut aminos)
- 1 teaspoon sesame oil (optional)

Instructions:
1. Set the Instant Pot to sauté mode and add the olive oil.
2. Add garlic and sauté for about 1 minute until fragrant.
3. Add shiitake mushrooms and sauté for about 3 minutes until they start to soften.
4. Add bok choy and soy sauce, and cook for another 3-5 minutes until the bok choy is wilted but still crisp.
5. Drizzle with sesame oil if using, stir to mix, and serve immediately.

Nutrition Info (Per Serving):
- Calories: 100
- Protein: 3g
- Fat: 7g
- Carbohydrates: 8g
- Fiber: 2g
- Serving Size: 4 servings
- Cooking Time: 10 minutes total

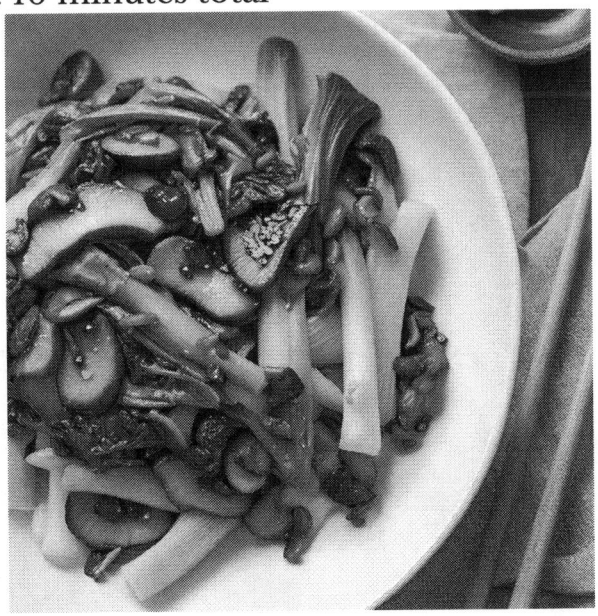

5. Basil Pesto Chicken Pasta

Ingredients:
- 1 pound chicken breast, cubed
- 2 cups pasta (gluten-free if needed)
- 1 cup homemade or store-bought low histamine pesto
- 2 cups water
- Salt to taste
- Fresh basil for garnish

Instructions:
1. Add chicken, pasta, pesto, and water to the Instant Pot.
2. Stir to make sure the pasta is fully submerged in the liquid.
3. Close the lid, set the valve to sealing, and cook on Manual High Pressure for 5 minutes.
4. Quick release the pressure after cooking is complete.
5. Stir well, adjust seasoning as needed, and garnish with fresh basil before serving.

Nutrition Info (Per Serving):
- Calories: 500
- Protein: 28g
- Fat: 22g
- Carbohydrates: 46g
- Fiber: 3g
- Serving Size: 4 servings
- Cooking Time: 15 minutes total

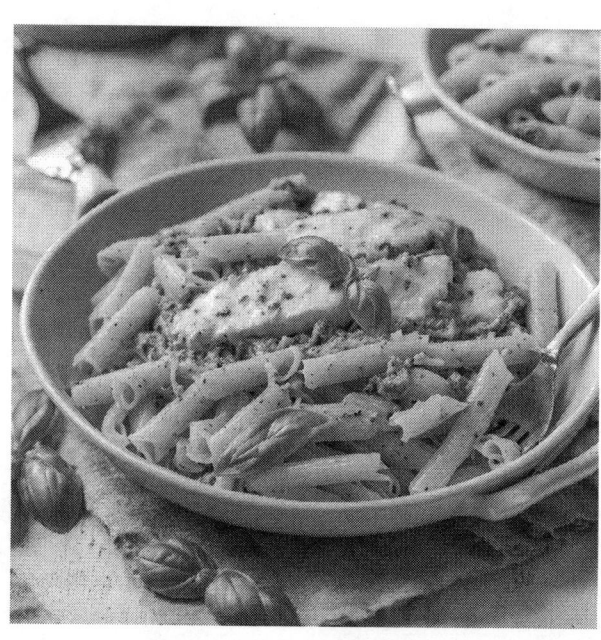

6. Carrot Ginger Soup

Ingredients:
- 2 tablespoons olive oil
- 1 onion, chopped
- 2 pounds carrots, peeled and chopped
- 2 tablespoons fresh ginger, minced
- 4 cups vegetable broth
- Salt and pepper to taste

Instructions:
1. Set the Instant Pot to sauté mode and heat the olive oil.
2. Add onion and ginger, and sauté until onion is translucent.
3. Add carrots and vegetable broth.
4. Close the lid, set the valve to sealing, and cook on Manual High Pressure for 15 minutes.
5. Quick release the pressure, then puree the soup using an immersion blender until smooth.
6. Season with salt and pepper, and serve hot.

Nutrition Info (Per Serving):
- Calories: 150
- Protein: 2g
- Fat: 7g
- Carbohydrates: 21g
- Fiber: 6g
- Serving Size: 4 servings
- Cooking Time: 25 minutes total

7. Turmeric Coconut Basmati Rice

Ingredients:
- 1 cup basmati rice, rinsed
- 1 3/4 cups coconut milk
- 1 teaspoon turmeric
- 1/2 teaspoon salt

Instructions:
1. Add the rinsed basmati rice, coconut milk, turmeric, and salt to the Instant Pot.
2. Stir to combine.
3. Close the lid, set the valve to sealing, and cook on the Rice setting (or Manual Low Pressure for 12 minutes).
4. Allow natural pressure release for 10 minutes, then quick release any remaining pressure.
5. Fluff the rice with a fork and serve.

Nutrition Info (Per Serving):
- Calories: 250
- Protein: 4g
- Fat: 14g
- Carbohydrates: 28g
- Fiber: 1g
- Serving Size: 4 servings
- Cooking Time: 22 minutes total

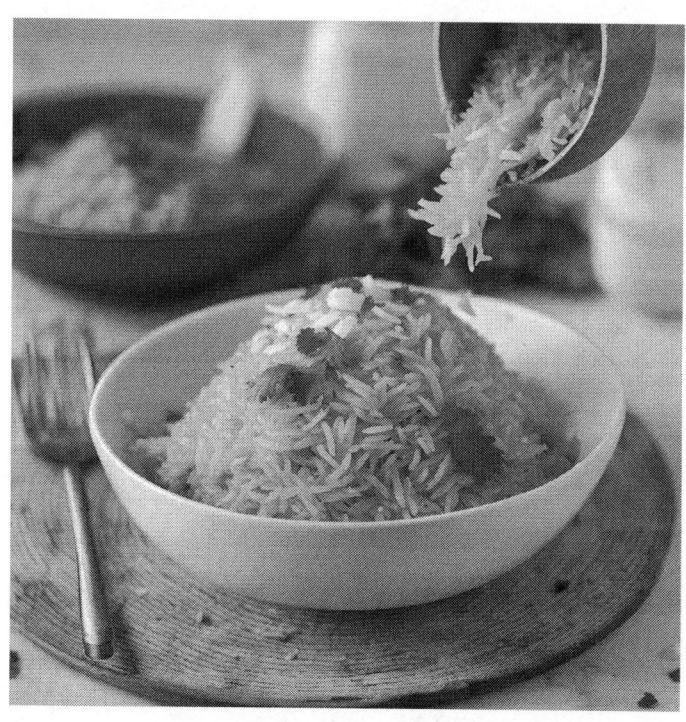

8. Zucchini Noodles with Olive Oil and Herbs

Ingredients:
- 4 medium zucchini, spiralized
- 2 tablespoons olive oil
- 1 clove garlic, minced
- 1 tablespoon fresh basil, chopped
- 1 tablespoon fresh parsley, chopped
- Salt and pepper to taste

Instructions:
1. Set the Instant Pot to sauté mode and add olive oil and garlic.
2. Sauté the garlic for 1 minute until fragrant.
3. Add the zucchini noodles and toss for about 2-3 minutes until just tender. Be careful not to overcook as they can become mushy.
4. Stir in basil and parsley, and season with salt and pepper.
5. Serve immediately.

Nutrition Info (Per Serving):
- Calories: 90
- Protein: 2g
- Fat: 7g
- Carbohydrates: 6g
- Fiber: 2g
- Serving Size: 4 servings
- Cooking Time: 5 minutes total

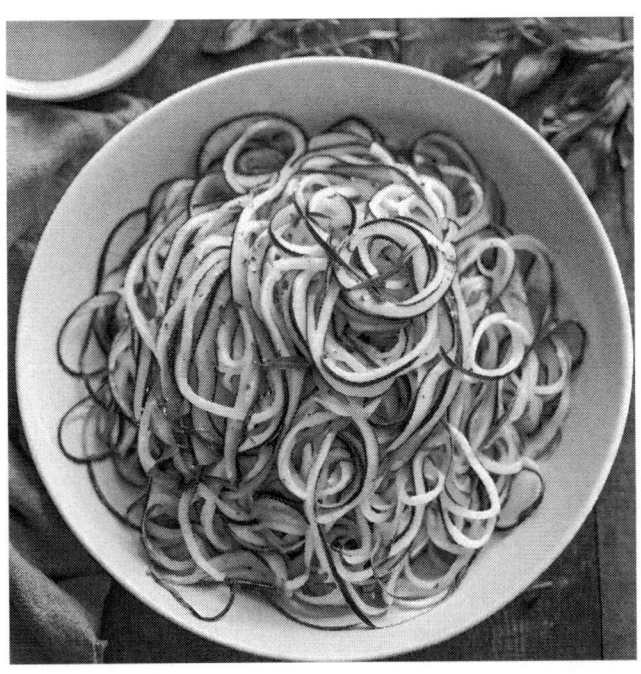

9. Beef Stew with Root Vegetables

Ingredients:
- 2 pounds beef stew meat, cut into cubes
- 1 tablespoon olive oil
- 1 onion, chopped
- 2 carrots, peeled and chopped
- 2 parsnips, peeled and chopped
- 3 cups beef broth
- 1 teaspoon thyme
- Salt and pepper to taste

Instructions:
1. Set the Instant Pot to sauté mode and heat the olive oil.
2. Brown the beef cubes in batches to ensure they sear properly.
3. Add the onion, carrots, and parsnips, and sauté for a few minutes.
4. Pour in the beef broth, add thyme, and season with salt and pepper.
5. Close the lid, set the valve to sealing, and cook on Manual High Pressure for 35 minutes.
6. Allow natural pressure release for 15 minutes, then quick release any remaining pressure.
7. Stir well before serving.

Nutrition Info (Per Serving):
- Calories: 380
- Protein: 35g
- Fat: 20g
- Carbohydrates: 15g
- Fiber: 3g
- Serving Size: 6 servings
- Cooking Time: 50 minutes total

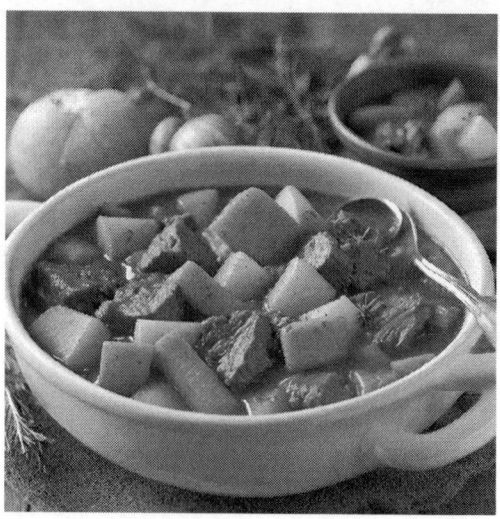

10. Stuffed Acorn Squash

Ingredients:
- 2 acorn squashes, halved and seeds removed
- 1 pound ground turkey
- 1 apple, chopped
- 1 onion, chopped
- 1 teaspoon sage
- 1/2 teaspoon thyme
- 1/2 cup breadcrumbs (gluten-free if necessary)
- Salt and pepper to taste
- 1 cup water

Instructions:
1. In a bowl, mix together ground turkey, apple, onion, sage, thyme, breadcrumbs, salt, and pepper.
2. Stuff the acorn squash halves with the turkey mixture.
3. Pour water into the Instant Pot and place the trivet inside.
4. Place the stuffed squash halves on the trivet.
5. Close the lid, set the valve to sealing, and cook on Manual High Pressure for 20 minutes.
6. Allow natural pressure release for 10 minutes, then quick release any remaining pressure.
7. Serve hot.

Nutrition Info (Per Serving):
- Calories: 315
- Protein: 22g
- Fat: 15g
- Carbohydrates: 25g
- Fiber: 5g
- Serving Size: 4 servings
- Cooking Time: 30 minutes total

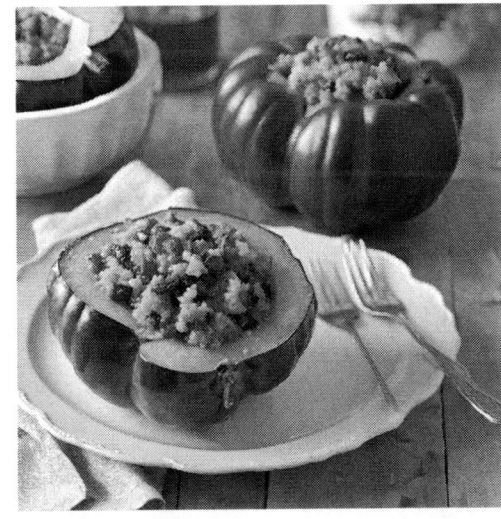

11. Rosemary Infused Lamb Stew

Ingredients:
- 2 pounds lamb stew meat, cubed
- 1 tablespoon olive oil
- 1 onion, chopped
- 3 carrots, peeled and sliced
- 2 cups beef or lamb broth
- 2 tablespoons fresh rosemary, chopped
- Salt and pepper to taste

Instructions:
1. Set the Instant Pot to sauté mode and heat the olive oil.
2. Brown the lamb cubes on all sides.
3. Add onion and carrots, and sauté for a few minutes.
4. Pour in the broth, add rosemary, and season with salt and pepper.
5. Close the lid, set the valve to sealing, and cook on Manual High Pressure for 30 minutes.
6. Allow natural pressure release for 15 minutes, then quick release any remaining pressure.
7. Stir well and serve hot.

Nutrition Info (Per Serving):
- Calories: 350
- Protein: 32g
- Fat: 20g
- Carbohydrates: 10g
- Fiber: 2g
- Serving Size: 6 servings
- Cooking Time: 45 minutes total

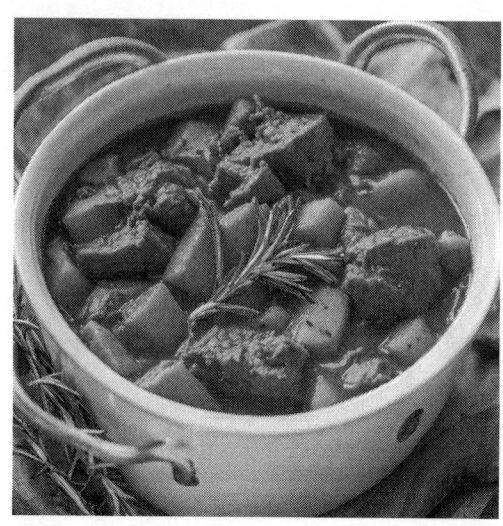

12. Instant Pot Fennel Chicken

Ingredients:
- 4 chicken breasts
- 1 fennel bulb, sliced
- 1 onion, sliced
- 3 cloves garlic, minced
- 1 lemon, sliced
- 1 cup chicken broth
- 1 teaspoon dried thyme
- Salt and pepper to taste
- 2 tablespoons olive oil

Instructions:
1. Set the Instant Pot to sauté mode and add olive oil.
2. Add garlic, onion, and fennel. Sauté for 3-5 minutes until slightly softened.
3. Season chicken breasts with salt, pepper, and thyme. Place them in the pot.
4. Top with sliced lemon.
5. Pour in the chicken broth.
6. Close the lid, set the valve to sealing, and cook on Manual High Pressure for 12 minutes.
7. Allow natural pressure release for 10 minutes, then quick release any remaining pressure.
8. Serve the chicken with fennel and onions, garnished with additional fresh herbs if desired.

Nutrition Info (Per Serving):
- Calories: 290
- Protein: 26g
- Fat: 15g
- Carbohydrates: 10g
- Fiber: 3g
- Serving Size: 4 servings
- Cooking Time: 27 minutes total

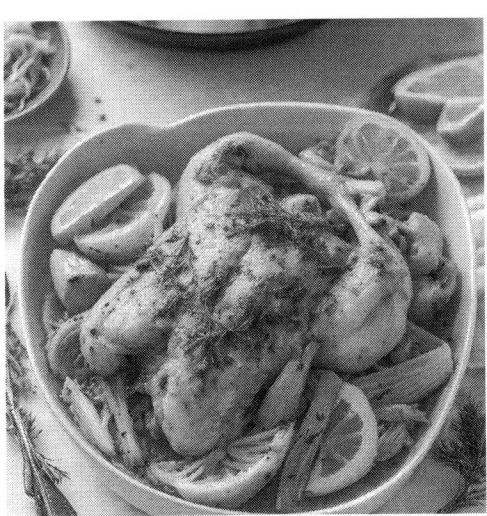

13. Golden Beet Soup

Ingredients:
- 2 pounds golden beets, peeled and chopped
- 1 onion, chopped
- 2 cloves garlic, minced
- 4 cups vegetable broth
- Salt and pepper to taste
- 2 tablespoons olive oil
- Fresh dill for garnish

Instructions:
1. Set the Instant Pot to sauté mode and heat the olive oil.
2. Add onion and garlic, sautéing until onion is translucent.
3. Add chopped beets and vegetable broth.
4. Close the lid, set the valve to sealing, and cook on Manual High Pressure for 15 minutes.
5. Quick release the pressure, then blend the soup using an immersion blender until smooth.
6. Season with salt and pepper.
7. Serve hot, garnished with fresh dill.

Nutrition Info (Per Serving):
- Calories: 180
- Protein: 4g
- Fat: 7g
- Carbohydrates: 27g
- Fiber: 6g
- Serving Size: 4 servings
- Cooking Time: 25 minutes total

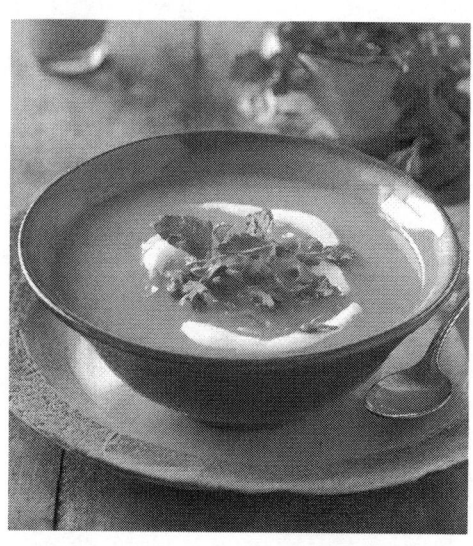

14. Sage and Butter Turkey Breast

Ingredients:
- 1 turkey breast (about 3 pounds)
- 1/4 cup butter, softened
- 2 tablespoons fresh sage, minced
- 2 cloves garlic, minced
- Salt and pepper to taste
- 1 cup chicken broth

Instructions:
1. Combine softened butter, minced sage, garlic, salt, and pepper in a bowl.
2. Rub the butter mixture all over the turkey breast.
3. Pour chicken broth into the Instant Pot and place the trivet inside.
4. Set the turkey breast on the trivet.
5. Close the lid, set the valve to sealing, and cook on Manual High Pressure for 25 minutes.
6. Allow natural pressure release for 20 minutes, then quick release any remaining pressure.
7. Let the turkey rest before slicing and serve with the juices from the pot.

Nutrition Info (Per Serving):
- Calories: 320
- Protein: 45g
- Fat: 14g
- Carbohydrates: 1g
- Fiber: 0g
- Serving Size: 6 servings
- Cooking Time: 45 minutes total

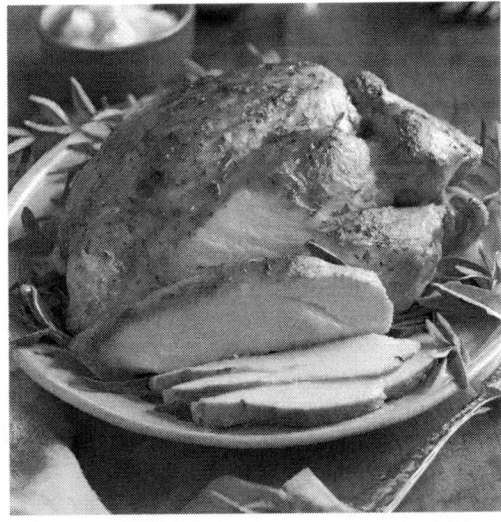

15. Instant Pot Cabbage Rolls

Ingredients:
- 12 cabbage leaves
- 1 pound ground turkey
- 1/2 cup cooked rice
- 1 onion, finely chopped
- 1 egg, beaten
- 2 cloves garlic, minced
- 1 can (14 oz) crushed tomatoes
- Salt and pepper to taste
- 1 teaspoon paprika

Instructions:
1. Blanch cabbage leaves in boiling water for 2 minutes to soften. Drain and set aside.
2. Mix ground turkey, cooked rice, onion, egg, garlic, salt, pepper, and paprika in a bowl.
3. Place a portion of the filling onto each cabbage leaf and roll tightly, tucking in the ends.
4. Pour half of the crushed tomatoes into the Instant Pot.
5. Arrange the cabbage rolls seam-side down in the pot.
6. Top with the remaining crushed tomatoes.
7. Close the lid, set the valve to sealing, and cook on Manual High Pressure for 15 minutes.
8. Quick release the pressure and serve the cabbage rolls hot.

Nutrition Info (Per Serving):
- Calories: 250
- Protein: 20g
- Fat: 10g
- Carbohydrates: 20g
- Fiber: 4g
- Serving Size: 6 servings
- Cooking Time: 30 minutes total

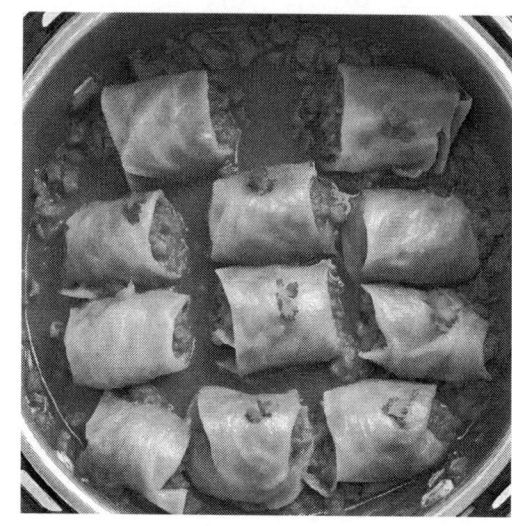

16. Lemon-Dill Salmon Steaks

Ingredients:
- 4 salmon steaks (about 6 ounces each)
- Juice of 1 lemon
- 2 tablespoons fresh dill, chopped
- Salt and pepper to taste
- 1 cup water

Instructions:
1. Season the salmon steaks with salt, pepper, lemon juice, and dill.
2. Pour water into the Instant Pot and insert the steam rack.
3. Place the salmon steaks on the rack.
4. Close the lid, set the valve to sealing, and cook on Manual High Pressure for 3 minutes.
5. Quick release the pressure immediately after cooking.
6. Serve the salmon steaks hot, garnished with additional dill and lemon slices if desired.

Nutrition Info (Per Serving):
- Calories: 250
- Protein: 34g
- Fat: 12g
- Carbohydrates: 0g
- Fiber: 0g
- Serving Size: 4 servings
- Cooking Time: 8 minutes total

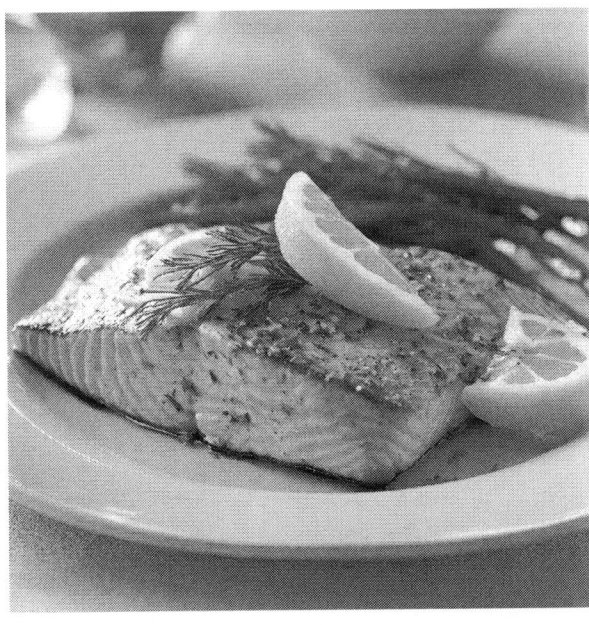

17. Root Vegetable Medley

Ingredients:
- 2 carrots, peeled and sliced
- 2 parsnips, peeled and sliced
- 1 sweet potato, peeled and cubed
- 1 turnip, peeled and cubed
- 2 tablespoons olive oil
- 1 teaspoon rosemary, chopped
- Salt and pepper to taste
- 1/2 cup water

Instructions:
1. Combine all the vegetables in a large bowl with olive oil, rosemary, salt, and pepper.
2. Pour water into the Instant Pot and place the steam rack inside.
3. Spread the vegetable mixture evenly on the rack.
4. Close the lid, set the valve to sealing, and cook on Manual High Pressure for 4 minutes.
5. Quick release the pressure after cooking.
6. Toss the vegetables before serving to distribute the flavors evenly.

Nutrition Info (Per Serving):
- Calories: 140
- Protein: 2g
- Fat: 7g
- Carbohydrates: 18g
- Fiber: 4g
- Serving Size: 4 servings
- Cooking Time: 9 minutes total

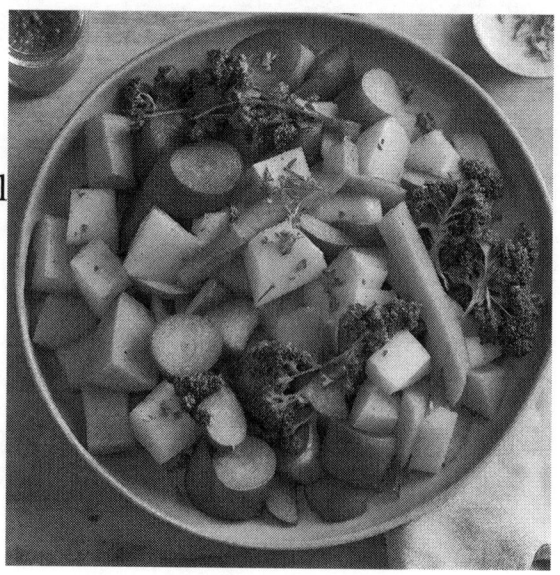

18. Parsley-Garlic Pork Chops

Ingredients:
- 4 pork chops (about 1-inch thick)
- 4 cloves garlic, minced
- 1/4 cup fresh parsley, chopped
- 2 tablespoons olive oil
- Salt and pepper to taste
- 1 cup chicken broth

Instructions:
1. Rub the pork chops with garlic, parsley, salt, and pepper.
2. Set the Instant Pot to sauté mode and heat the olive oil.
3. Brown the pork chops on both sides.
4. Add chicken broth to the pot.
5. Close the lid, set the valve to sealing, and cook on Manual High Pressure for 10 minutes.
6. Allow natural pressure release for 5 minutes, then quick release any remaining pressure.
7. Serve the pork chops with a garnish of extra parsley.

Nutrition Info (Per Serving):
- Calories: 300
- Protein: 25g
- Fat: 20g
- Carbohydrates: 2g
- Fiber: 0g
- Serving Size: 4 servings
- Cooking Time: 20 minutes total

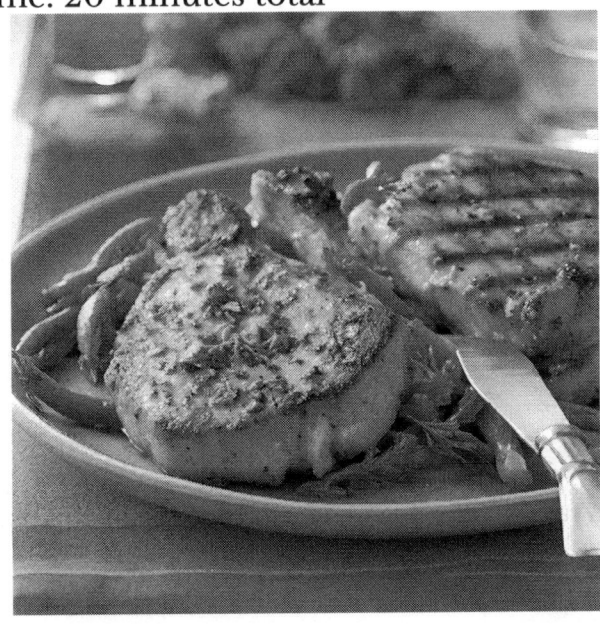

19. Instant Pot Spiced Apple Cider Chicken

Ingredients:
- 4 chicken breasts
- 1 cup apple cider
- 1 onion, sliced
- 2 cloves garlic, minced
- 1 teaspoon cinnamon
- 1/2 teaspoon allspice
- Salt and pepper to taste
- 2 tablespoons olive oil

Instructions:
1. Season the chicken breasts with cinnamon, allspice, salt, and pepper.
2. Set the Instant Pot to sauté mode and heat the olive oil.
3. Brown the chicken and garlic briefly on both sides.
4. Add the onion and apple cider.
5. Close the lid, set the valve to sealing, and cook on Manual High Pressure for 8 minutes.
6. Quick release the pressure after cooking.
7. Serve the chicken topped with the cider and onion sauce.

Nutrition Info (Per Serving):
- Calories: 230 Protein: 26g Fat: 9g Carbohydrates: 10g
- Fiber: 1g
- Serving Size: 4 servings
- Cooking Time: 18 minutes total

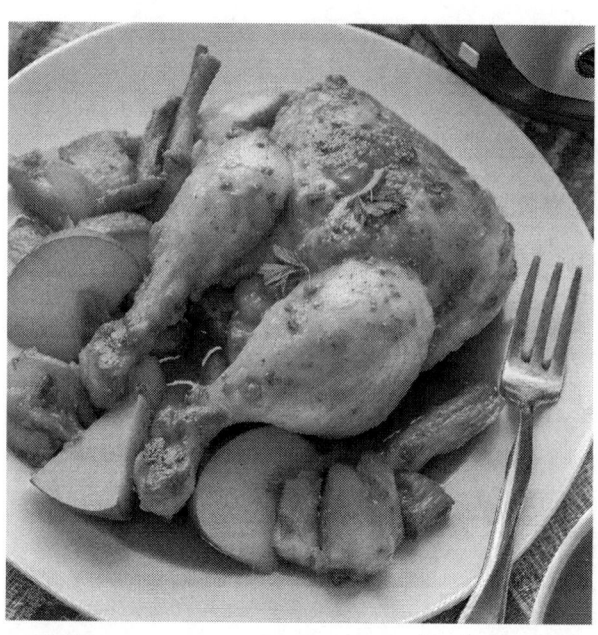

20. Saffron Vegetable Couscous

Ingredients:
- 1 cup couscous
- 1 1/4 cups vegetable broth
- A pinch of saffron threads
- 1 cup mixed vegetables (carrots, zucchini, bell peppers), chopped
- 1 tablespoon olive oil
- Salt to taste

Instructions:
1. Soak the saffron threads in a few tablespoons of warm water for about 10 minutes.
2. Set the Instant Pot to sauté mode and heat the olive oil.
3. Sauté the mixed vegetables for about 5 minutes until they begin to soften.
4. Add the couscous, vegetable broth, saffron with its soaking liquid, and salt.
5. Stir to combine all the ingredients.
6. Close the lid, set the valve to sealing, and switch to the Manual Low Pressure setting for 1 minute.
7. Quick release the pressure as soon as the cooking time is complete.
8. Fluff the couscous with a fork and serve warm.

Nutrition Info (Per Serving):
- Calories: 220 Protein: 6g Fat: 4g Carbohydrates: 40g
- Fiber: 3g
- Serving Size: 4 servings
- Cooking Time: 16 minutes total

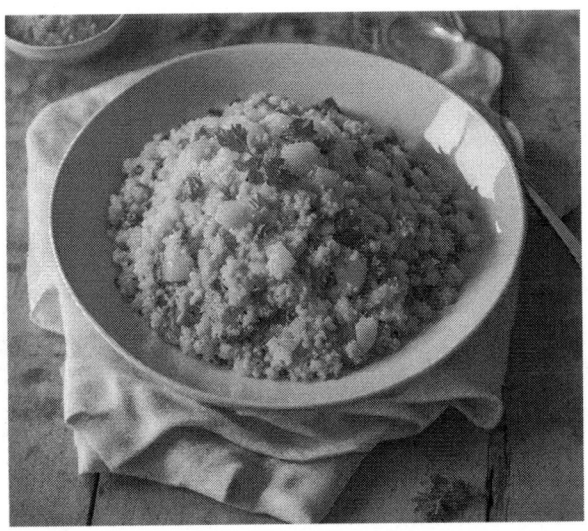

21. Herbed Quinoa and Vegetable Stuffed Peppers

Ingredients:
- 4 bell peppers, tops cut off and seeds removed
- 1 cup quinoa, rinsed
- 2 cups vegetable broth
- 1 zucchini, diced
- 1 carrot, diced
- 1/2 onion, diced
- 1 tablespoon olive oil
- 1 teaspoon dried basil
- 1 teaspoon dried oregano
- Salt and pepper to taste

Instructions:
1. Set the Instant Pot to sauté mode and heat the olive oil.
2. Add onion, carrot, and zucchini. Sauté until vegetables are slightly softened, about 5 minutes.
3. Add quinoa, vegetable broth, basil, oregano, salt, and pepper. Stir to combine.
4. Stuff the bell peppers with the quinoa and vegetable mixture.
5. Pour one cup of water into the Instant Pot and place the stuffed peppers on the trivet.
6. Close the lid, set the valve to sealing, and cook on Manual High Pressure for 8 minutes.
7. Quick release the pressure after cooking.
8. Serve the stuffed peppers hot, garnished with fresh herbs if desired.

Nutrition Info (Per Serving):
- Calories: 250
- Protein: 8g
- Fat: 7g
- Carbohydrates: 40g
- Fiber: 6g
- Serving Size: 4 servings
- Cooking Time: 20 minutes total

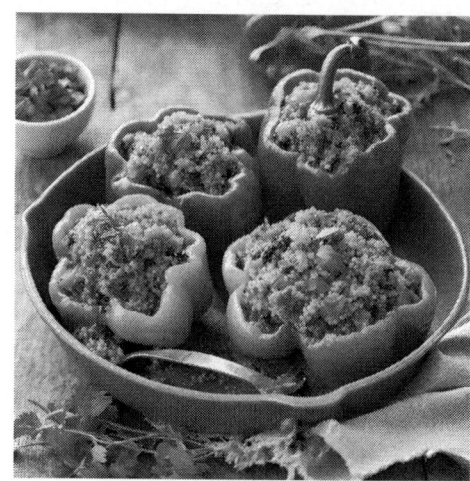

22. Instant Pot Maple-Glazed Chicken

Ingredients:
- 4 chicken breasts
- 1/2 cup maple syrup
- 2 tablespoons soy sauce (or coconut aminos for low histamine)
- 1 tablespoon Dijon mustard
- 1 tablespoon olive oil
- Salt and pepper to taste

Instructions:
1. Season the chicken breasts with salt and pepper.
2. Mix the maple syrup, soy sauce, and Dijon mustard in a bowl.
3. Set the Instant Pot to sauté mode and heat the olive oil.
4. Brown the chicken on both sides.
5. Pour the maple syrup mixture over the chicken.
6. Close the lid, set the valve to sealing, and cook on Manual High Pressure for 10 minutes.
7. Quick release the pressure after cooking.
8. Serve the chicken drizzled with the glaze from the pot.

Nutrition Info (Per Serving):
- Calories: 320
- Protein: 26g
- Fat: 8g
- Carbohydrates: 34g
- Fiber: 0g
- Serving Size: 4 servings
- Cooking Time: 20 minutes total

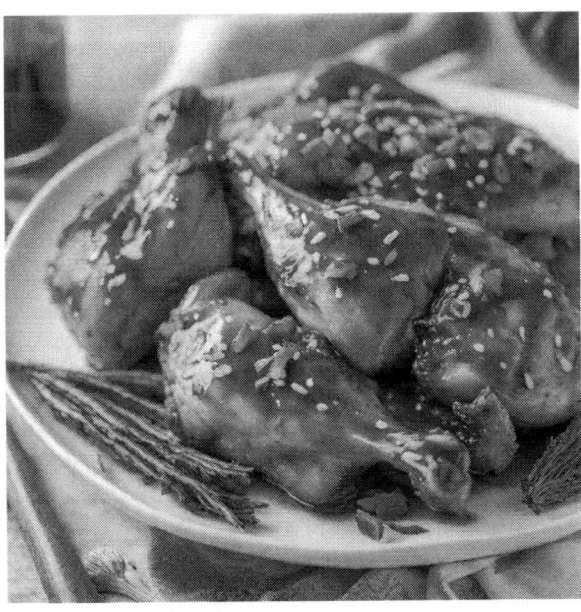

23. Instant Pot Tarragon Chicken

Ingredients:
- 4 chicken thighs, bone-in, skin-on
- 1 tablespoon dried tarragon
- 1/2 cup chicken broth
- 2 tablespoons lemon juice
- 1 tablespoon olive oil
- Salt and pepper to taste

Instructions:
1. Season chicken thighs with salt, pepper, and tarragon.
2. Set the Instant Pot to sauté mode and heat the olive oil.
3. Brown the chicken thighs, skin-side down first, until golden.
4. Flip the chicken, add lemon juice and chicken broth.
5. Close the lid, set the valve to sealing, and cook on Manual High Pressure for 15 minutes.
6. Natural release for 10 minutes, then quick release any remaining pressure.
7. Serve the chicken garnished with additional tarragon and a splash of the cooking liquid.

Nutrition Info (Per Serving):
- Calories: 310
- Protein: 24g
- Fat: 22g
- Carbohydrates: 1g
- Fiber: 0g
- Serving Size: 4 servings
- Cooking Time: 30 minutes total

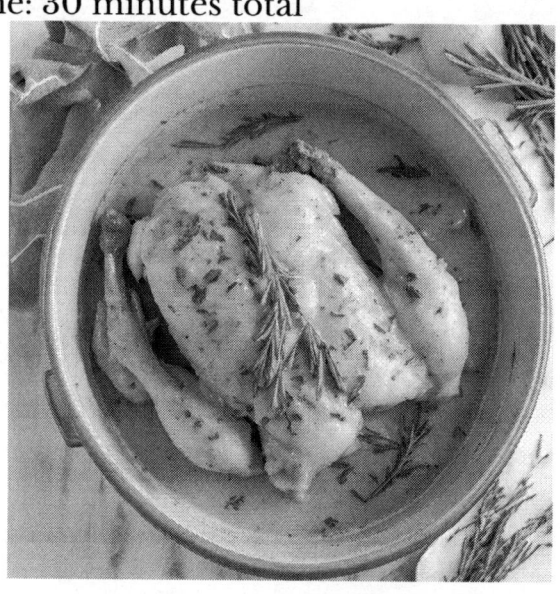

24. Lemon-Basil Shrimp Over Zoodles

Ingredients:
- 1 pound large shrimp, peeled and deveined
- Juice and zest of 1 lemon
- 2 tablespoons fresh basil, chopped
- 2 cloves garlic, minced
- 2 tablespoons olive oil
- Salt and pepper to taste
- 4 medium zucchini, spiralized into noodles

Instructions:
1. In a bowl, toss the shrimp with lemon zest, minced garlic, salt, and pepper.
2. Set the Instant Pot to sauté mode and heat 1 tablespoon of olive oil.
3. Add the shrimp and sauté until they are pink and opaque, about 3-4 minutes. Remove shrimp and set aside.
4. In the same pot, add the remaining tablespoon of olive oil. Add the zucchini noodles and sauté for about 2 minutes, just until tender.
5. Turn off the Instant Pot, add the shrimp back to the pot along with the fresh basil and lemon juice, and toss to combine.
6. Serve immediately, ensuring not to overcook the zoodles to keep them crisp.

Nutrition Info (Per Serving):
- Calories: 230
- Protein: 24g
- Fat: 12g
- Carbohydrates: 6g
- Fiber: 2g
- Serving Size: 4 servings
- Cooking Time: 10 minutes total

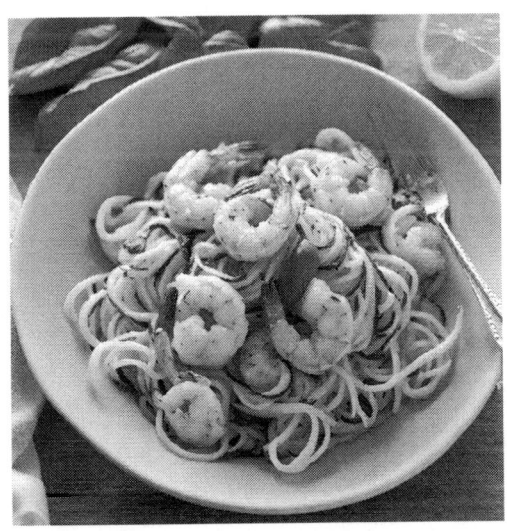

25. Instant Pot Moroccan Vegetable Tagine
Ingredients:
- 1 tablespoon olive oil
- 1 onion, chopped
- 2 cloves garlic, minced
- 1 sweet potato, cubed
- 1 carrot, sliced
- 1 bell pepper, chopped
- 1 zucchini, chopped
- 1 can (14 oz) diced tomatoes
- 1 teaspoon cumin
- 1 teaspoon coriander
- 1/2 teaspoon cinnamon
- 1/2 cup vegetable broth
- Salt and pepper to taste
- Fresh cilantro for garnish

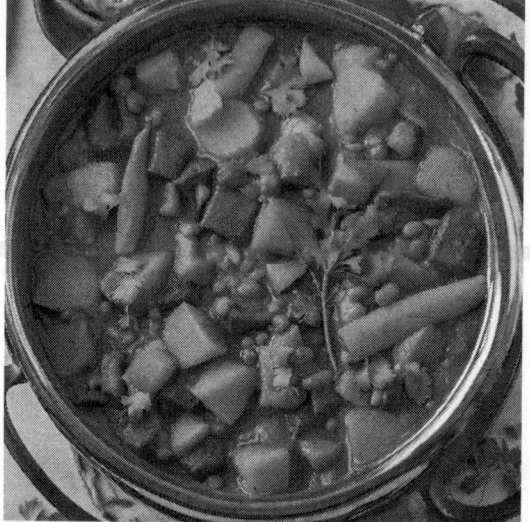

Instructions:
1. Set the Instant Pot to sauté mode and heat the olive oil.
2. Add onion and garlic, and sauté until soft.
3. Add sweet potato, carrot, bell pepper, and zucchini, cooking for a few minutes until slightly softened.
4. Stir in the spices and diced tomatoes.
5. Pour in the vegetable broth and season with salt and pepper.
6. Close the lid, set the valve to sealing, and cook on Manual High Pressure for 5 minutes.
7. Quick release the pressure when cooking is complete.
8. Serve the tagine garnished with fresh cilantro.

Nutrition Info (Per Serving):
- Calories: 150
- Protein: 3g
- Fat: 4g
- Carbohydrates: 27g
- Fiber: 6g
- Serving Size: 4 servings
- Cooking Time: 20 minutes total

26. Garlic-Infused Olive Oil Drizzled Cod

Ingredients:
- 4 cod fillets (about 6 ounces each)
- 2 tablespoons olive oil
- 4 cloves garlic, minced
- Juice of 1 lemon
- Salt and pepper to taste
- 1/2 cup water

Instructions:
1. In a small bowl, mix olive oil and minced garlic. Let sit for at least 30 minutes to infuse the flavor.
2. Season the cod fillets with salt and pepper and drizzle with half of the garlic-infused olive oil.
3. Pour water into the Instant Pot and place the steam rack inside.
4. Place the cod fillets on the rack.
5. Close the lid, set the valve to sealing, and cook on Manual High Pressure for 2 minutes.
6. Quick release the pressure immediately after cooking.
7. Drizzle the remaining garlic-infused olive oil and lemon juice over the cod before serving.

Nutrition Info (Per Serving):
- Calories: 180
- Protein: 23g
- Fat: 9g
- Carbohydrates: 1g
- Fiber: 0g
- Serving Size: 4 servings
- Cooking Time: 7 minutes total

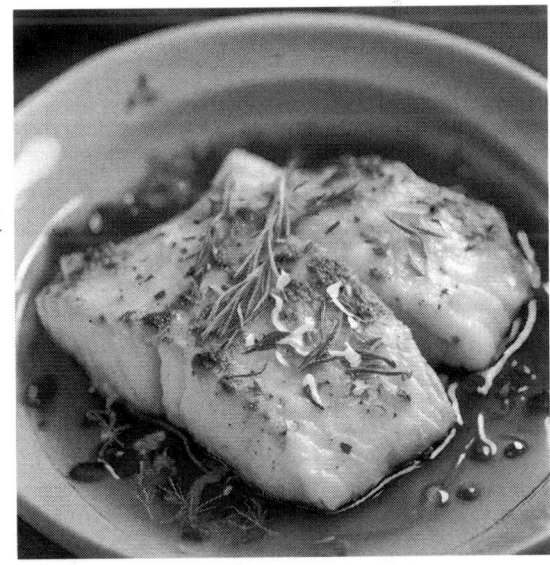

DESSERTS

1. Sticky Ginger Pudding
Ingredients:
- 1 cup all-purpose flour
- 1/2 cup dark brown sugar
- 1 tablespoon ground ginger
- 1 teaspoon baking soda
- 1/2 cup milk
- 1/4 cup molasses
- 1/4 cup melted butter
- 1 egg, beaten
- 1 cup hot water
- 3/4 cup additional dark brown sugar

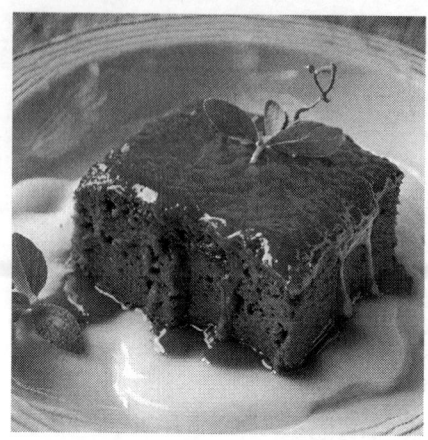

Instructions:
1. In a bowl, mix flour, 1/2 cup brown sugar, ginger, and baking soda.
2. Stir in milk, molasses, melted butter, and beaten egg until smooth.
3. Pour the batter into a greased cake pan that fits inside your Instant Pot.
4. Mix hot water and 3/4 cup brown sugar until dissolved and pour over the batter.
5. Cover the cake pan tightly with foil.
6. Pour 1 cup of water into the Instant Pot and place the trivet. Set the cake pan on the trivet.
7. Close the lid, set the valve to sealing, and cook on Manual High Pressure for 30 minutes.
8. Allow natural pressure release for 10 minutes, then quick release any remaining pressure.
9. Carefully remove the cake and serve warm.

Nutrition Info (Per Serving):
- Calories: 320 Protein: 3g Fat: 11g Carbohydrates: 54g
- Fiber: 1g
- Serving Size: 6 servings
- Cooking Time: 40 minutes total

2. Maple Blondies

Ingredients:
- 1/2 cup unsalted butter, melted
- 1 cup all-purpose flour
- 1 cup brown sugar
- 1/2 cup maple syrup
- 1 egg
- 1 teaspoon vanilla extract
- 1/2 teaspoon baking powder
- 1/4 teaspoon salt
- 1/2 cup chopped walnuts (optional)

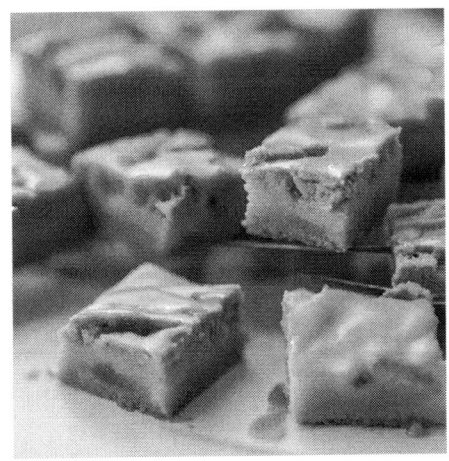

Instructions:
1. In a bowl, combine melted butter, brown sugar, maple syrup, and vanilla extract. Beat in the egg.
2. Mix in flour, baking powder, salt, and walnuts until well combined.
3. Pour the mixture into a greased cake pan that fits in your Instant Pot.
4. Pour 1 cup of water into the Instant Pot and place the trivet. Set the cake pan on the trivet.
5. Cover the cake pan with foil.
6. Close the lid, set the valve to sealing, and cook on Manual High Pressure for 40 minutes.
7. Quick release the pressure after cooking.
8. Let the blondies cool before slicing and serving.

Nutrition Info (Per Serving):
- Calories: 330
- Protein: 3g
- Fat: 15g
- Carbohydrates: 46g
- Fiber: 1g
- Serving Size: 8 servings
- Cooking Time: 50 minutes total

3. Vanilla Rice Pudding

Ingredients:
- 1 cup Arborio rice
- 4 cups milk
- 1/2 cup sugar
- 1 vanilla bean, split lengthwise (or 1 teaspoon vanilla extract)
- Pinch of salt

Instructions:
1. Combine rice, milk, sugar, vanilla bean, and salt in the Instant Pot.
2. Stir well to mix the ingredients.
3. Close the lid, set the valve to sealing, and cook on the Porridge setting or Manual Low Pressure for 20 minutes.
4. Allow natural pressure release for 10 minutes, then quick release any remaining pressure.
5. Remove the vanilla bean, scrape out the seeds, and stir back into the pudding.
6. Serve warm or chilled, garnished with cinnamon or nutmeg if desired.

Nutrition Info (Per Serving):
- Calories: 215
- Protein: 5g
- Fat: 3g
- Carbohydrates: 40g
- Fiber: 1g
- Serving Size: 6 servings
- Cooking Time: 30 minutes total

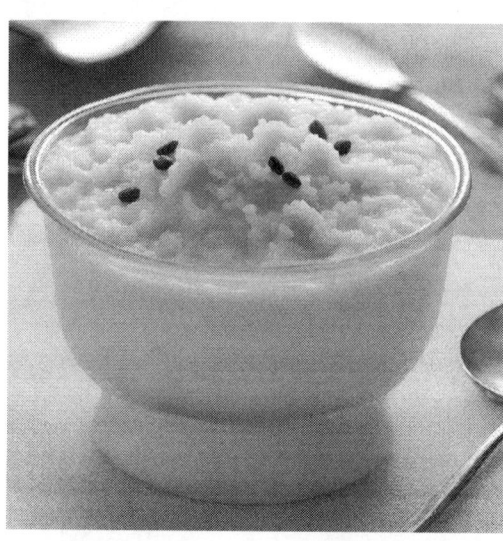

4. Maple-Poached Pears

Ingredients:
- 4 pears, peeled, halved, and cored
- 1 cup maple syrup
- 2 cups water
- 1 cinnamon stick
- 1 vanilla bean, split (or 1 teaspoon vanilla extract)

Instructions:
1. Combine maple syrup, water, cinnamon stick, and vanilla bean in the Instant Pot.
2. Add the pear halves.
3. Close the lid, set the valve to sealing, and cook on Manual High Pressure for 5 minutes.
4. Quick release the pressure immediately after cooking.
5. Carefully remove the pears and serve them warm with a drizzle of the cooking syrup.

Nutrition Info (Per Serving):
- Calories: 290
- Protein: 1g
- Fat: 0g
- Carbohydrates: 76g
- Fiber: 6g
- Serving Size: 4 servings
- Cooking Time: 10 minutes total

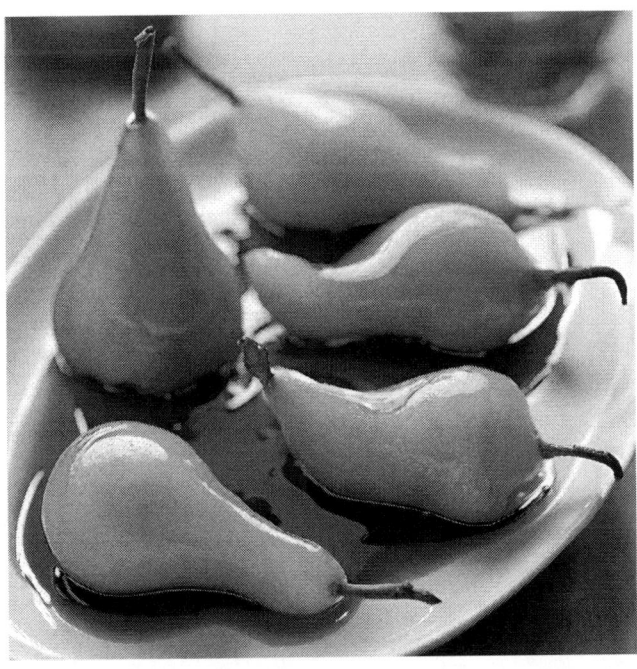

5. Coconut Custard

Ingredients:
- 4 eggs
- 1/3 cup sugar
- 1 can (14 oz) coconut milk
- 1 teaspoon vanilla extract
- Pinch of salt

Instructions:
1. Whisk together eggs, sugar, coconut milk, vanilla extract, and salt in a bowl until smooth.
2. Pour the mixture into a heat-proof dish that will fit in your Instant Pot.
3. Pour 1 cup of water into the Instant Pot and place the trivet inside.
4. Set the dish on the trivet.
5. Close the lid, set the valve to sealing, and cook on Manual Low Pressure for 10 minutes.
6. Allow natural pressure release for 10 minutes, then quick release any remaining pressure.
7. Chill the custard in the refrigerator before serving.

Nutrition Info (Per Serving):
- Calories: 250
- Protein: 6g
- Fat: 20g
- Carbohydrates: 14g
- Fiber: 0g
- Serving Size: 4 servings
- Cooking Time: 20 minutes total

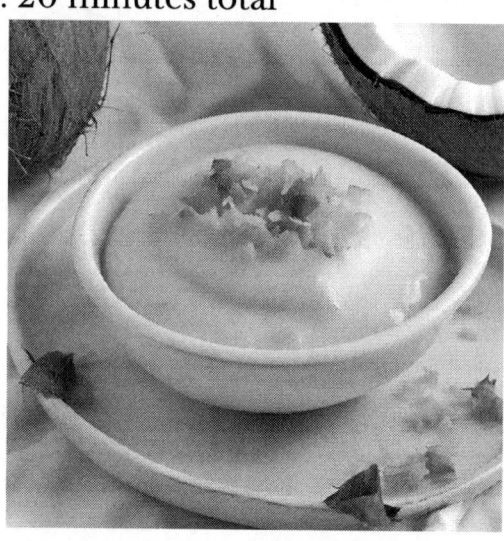

6. Ginger Poached Rhubarb

Ingredients:
- 4 cups rhubarb, cut into 1-inch pieces
- 1/2 cup sugar
- 1 cup water
- 2 tablespoons fresh ginger, grated
- 1 vanilla bean, split (or 1 teaspoon vanilla extract)

Instructions:
1. Combine water, sugar, ginger, and vanilla bean in the Instant Pot and stir until sugar dissolves.
2. Add the rhubarb pieces.
3. Close the lid, set the valve to sealing, and cook on Manual High Pressure for 1 minute.
4. Quick release the pressure immediately after cooking.
5. Serve the rhubarb warm or chilled, with a bit of the poaching liquid drizzled over the top.

Nutrition Info (Per Serving):
- Calories: 130
- Protein: 1g
- Fat: 0g
- Carbohydrates: 31g
- Fiber: 3g
- Serving Size: 4 servings
- Cooking Time: 6 minutes total

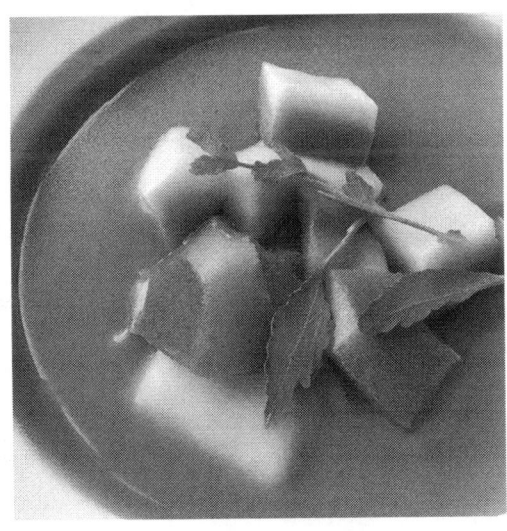

7. Pumpkin Spice Cake

Ingredients:
- 1 1/2 cups all-purpose flour
- 1 cup sugar
- 1/2 cup vegetable oil
- 2 eggs
- 1 cup pumpkin puree
- 1 teaspoon baking soda
- 1 teaspoon cinnamon
- 1/2 teaspoon nutmeg
- 1/4 teaspoon cloves
- 1/2 teaspoon salt

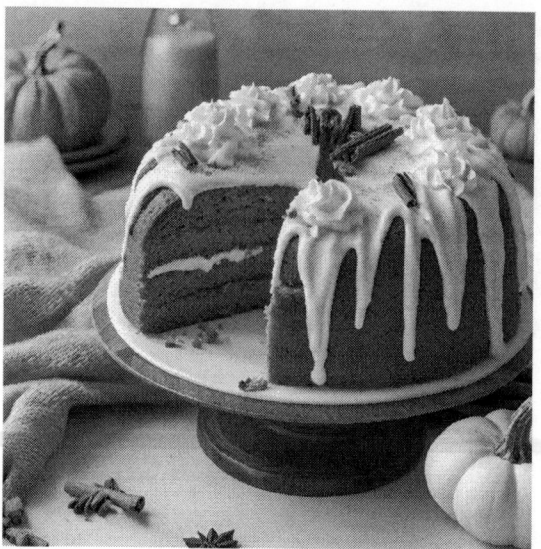

Instructions:
1. Mix together flour, sugar, baking soda, cinnamon, nutmeg, cloves, and salt in a bowl.
2. In another bowl, combine oil, eggs, and pumpkin puree.
3. Stir the wet ingredients into the dry until well mixed.
4. Pour the batter into a greased cake pan that fits in your Instant Pot.
5. Pour 1 cup of water into the Instant Pot and place the trivet inside.
6. Set the cake pan on the trivet.
7. Close the lid, set the valve to sealing, and cook on Manual High Pressure for 50 minutes.
8. Allow natural pressure release for 10 minutes, then quick release any remaining pressure.
9. Let the cake cool before serving.

Nutrition Info (Per Serving):
- Calories: 320
- Protein: 4g
- Fat: 15g
- Carbohydrates: 42g
- Fiber: 2g
- Serving Size: 8 servings
- Cooking Time: 60 minutes total

8. Instant Pot Berry Compote

Ingredients:
- 4 cups mixed berries (fresh or frozen)
- 1/2 cup sugar
- Juice of 1 lemon

Instructions:
1. Combine berries, sugar, and lemon juice in the Instant Pot.
2. Close the lid, set the valve to sealing, and cook on Manual High Pressure for 1 minute.
3. Quick release the pressure immediately after cooking.
4. If desired, mash the berries slightly for a smoother texture or leave them chunky.
5. Serve the compote warm or chilled, perfect as a topping for yogurt, pancakes, or ice cream.

Nutrition Info (Per Serving):
- Calories: 100
- Protein: 1g
- Fat: 0g
- Carbohydrates: 25g
- Fiber: 3g
- Serving Size: 6 servings
- Cooking Time: 6 minutes total

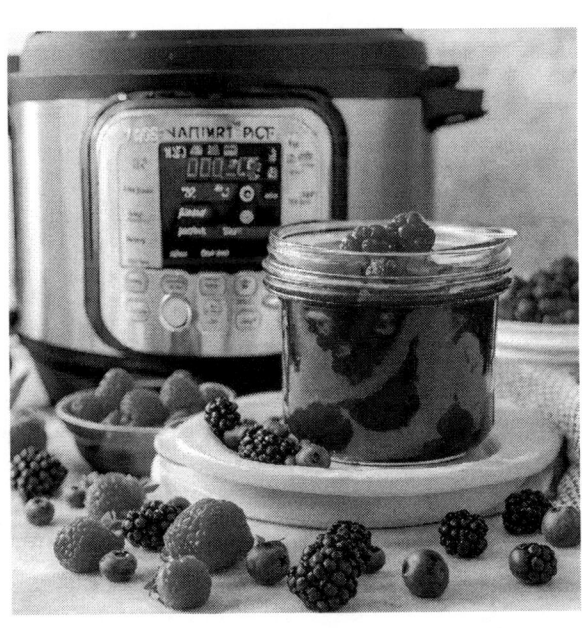

9. Peach Crumble

Ingredients:
- 4 peaches, peeled and sliced
- 1/2 cup rolled oats
- 1/2 cup almond flour
- 1/4 cup brown sugar
- 1/4 cup cold butter, cubed
- 1 teaspoon cinnamon
- 1/4 teaspoon nutmeg
- 1 cup water (for the Instant Pot)

Instructions:
1. In a bowl, mix together oats, almond flour, brown sugar, cinnamon, and nutmeg.
2. Cut in the butter until the mixture resembles coarse crumbs.
3. Place the sliced peaches in a greased heat-proof dish that fits inside your Instant Pot.
4. Sprinkle the oat mixture over the peaches.
5. Pour water into the Instant Pot and place the trivet inside. Place the dish on the trivet.
6. Close the lid, set the valve to sealing, and cook on Manual High Pressure for 8 minutes.
7. Quick release the pressure after cooking.
8. Optional: For a crispier top, place under a broiler for a few minutes before serving.

Nutrition Info (Per Serving):
- Calories: 220
- Protein: 3g
- Fat: 12g
- Carbohydrates: 26g
- Fiber: 4g
- Serving Size: 6 servings
- Cooking Time: 13 minutes total

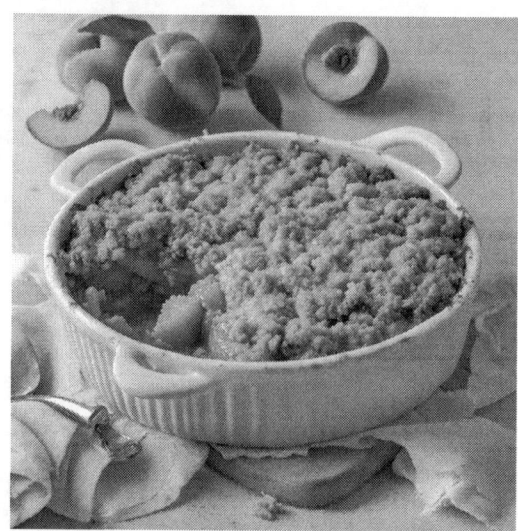

10. Mint and Lime Infused Mango

Ingredients:
- 2 large mangoes, peeled and cubed
- Juice of 2 limes
- 1/4 cup fresh mint leaves, chopped
- 1 tablespoon honey (optional)

Instructions:
1. In a bowl, combine mango cubes with lime juice, chopped mint, and honey if using.
2. Place the mango mixture in a heat-proof dish that fits inside your Instant Pot.
3. Pour 1 cup of water into the Instant Pot and place the trivet inside. Set the dish on the trivet.
4. Close the lid, set the valve to sealing, and cook on Manual Low Pressure for 2 minutes.
5. Quick release the pressure after cooking.
6. Chill before serving to allow flavors to meld.

Nutrition Info (Per Serving):
- Calories: 100
- Protein: 1g
- Fat: 0g
- Carbohydrates: 25g
- Fiber: 3g
- Serving Size: 4 servings
- Cooking Time: 7 minutes total

11. Cinnamon Applesauce

Ingredients:
- 6 large apples, peeled, cored, and chopped
- 1/2 cup water
- Juice of 1 lemon
- 2 teaspoons cinnamon
- 1/4 cup sugar (optional)

Instructions:
1. Combine all ingredients in the Instant Pot and stir well.
2. Close the lid, set the valve to sealing, and cook on Manual High Pressure for 8 minutes.
3. Quick release the pressure after cooking.
4. Mash the apples with a potato masher or blend with an immersion blender for a smoother texture.
5. Serve warm or chilled.

Nutrition Info (Per Serving):
- Calories: 150
- Protein: 0g
- Fat: 0g
- Carbohydrates: 40g
- Fiber: 6g
- Serving Size: 6 servings
- Cooking Time: 13 minutes total

12. Blueberry Flan

Ingredients:
- 1 cup blueberries (fresh or frozen)
- 3 eggs
- 1 can (14 oz) sweetened condensed milk
- 1 can (12 oz) evaporated milk
- 1 teaspoon vanilla extract
- 1/4 cup sugar (for caramel)

Instructions:
1. Pour sugar into a heat-proof dish suitable for the Instant Pot. Heat the dish on the stove or in the oven until sugar melts and becomes caramel. Swirl to coat the bottom of the dish.
2. Blend together eggs, sweetened condensed milk, evaporated milk, and vanilla until smooth.
3. Gently stir in blueberries.
4. Pour the mixture over the caramel in the dish.
5. Pour 1 cup of water into the Instant Pot and place the trivet inside. Set the dish on the trivet.
6. Close the lid, set the valve to sealing, and cook on Manual High Pressure for 20 minutes.
7. Allow natural pressure release for 10 minutes, then quick release any remaining pressure.
8. Chill before serving.

Nutrition Info (Per Serving):
- Calories: 320
- Protein: 9g
- Fat: 9g
- Carbohydrates: 51g
- Fiber: 1g
- Serving Size: 6 servings
- Cooking Time: 30 minutes total

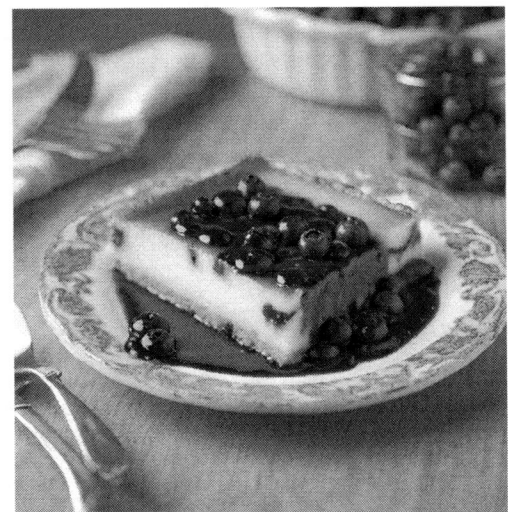

13. Saffron Poached Figs

Ingredients:
- 12 fresh figs, halved
- 1 cup water
- 1/4 cup honey
- A pinch of saffron threads
- 1 cinnamon stick

Instructions:
1. In the Instant Pot, combine water, honey, saffron, and the cinnamon stick. Stir to mix.
2. Add the fig halves to the pot, ensuring they are submerged in the liquid.
3. Close the lid, set the valve to sealing, and cook on Manual High Pressure for 2 minutes.
4. Quick release the pressure immediately after cooking.
5. Serve the figs warm, with a bit of the poaching liquid spooned over the top.

Nutrition Info (Per Serving):
- Calories: 110
- Protein: 1g
- Fat: 0.5g
- Carbohydrates: 28g
- Fiber: 4g
- Serving Size: 4 servings
- Cooking Time: 7 minutes total

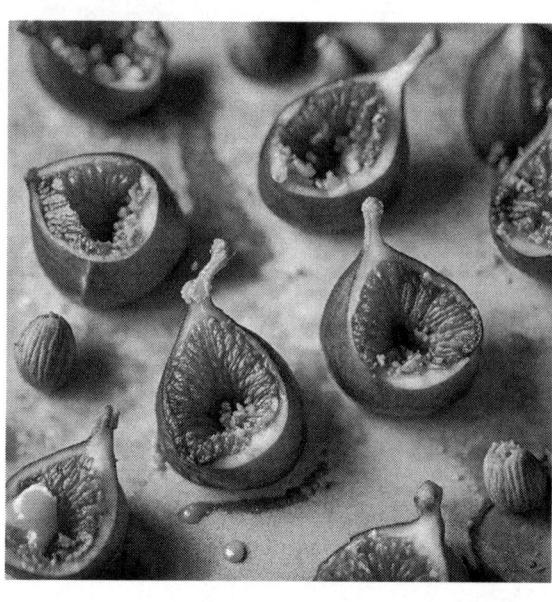

14. Pear and Ginger Jam

Ingredients:
- 4 large pears, peeled, cored, and finely chopped
- 1 cup sugar
- 2 tablespoons fresh ginger, grated
- Juice of 1 lemon

Instructions:
1. Combine all ingredients in the Instant Pot and stir to mix thoroughly.
2. Close the lid, set the valve to sealing, and cook on Manual High Pressure for 1 minute.
3. Use a quick release to depressurize.
4. If desired, use a potato masher or immersion blender to mash the jam to your preferred consistency.
5. Set the pot to sauté mode and cook for an additional 5-10 minutes to thicken the jam, stirring frequently.
6. Allow to cool, then store in sterilized jars. Refrigerate after sealing.

Nutrition Info (Per Serving):
- Calories: 150
- Protein: 0g
- Fat: 0g
- Carbohydrates: 38g
- Fiber: 3g
- Serving Size: 8 servings
- Cooking Time: 16 minutes total

15. Apple and Cranberry Crisp

Ingredients:
- 4 apples, peeled, cored, and sliced
- 1 cup fresh cranberries
- 1/2 cup rolled oats
- 1/2 cup almond flour
- 1/2 cup brown sugar
- 1/4 cup cold butter, cubed
- 1 teaspoon cinnamon
- 1/2 teaspoon nutmeg
- 1 cup water (for the Instant Pot)

Instructions:
1. In a bowl, combine apples and cranberries, and pour into a greased cake pan that fits in your Instant Pot.
2. In another bowl, mix oats, almond flour, brown sugar, cinnamon, and nutmeg. Cut in the butter until the mixture resembles coarse crumbs.
3. Sprinkle the crumb mixture over the fruit.
4. Pour water into the Instant Pot and place the trivet inside. Place the cake pan on the trivet.
5. Close the lid, set the valve to sealing, and cook on Manual High Pressure for 8 minutes.
6. Quick release the pressure after cooking.
7. Serve warm, ideally with a scoop of vanilla ice cream or a dollop of whipped cream.

Nutrition Info (Per Serving):
- Calories: 250
- Protein: 3g
- Fat: 12g
- Carbohydrates: 35g
- Fiber: 5g
- Serving Size: 6 servings
- Cooking Time: 13 minutes total

16. Banana Coconut Bread

Ingredients:
- 2 ripe bananas, mashed
- 1/3 cup melted coconut oil
- 1/2 cup coconut sugar
- 2 eggs, beaten
- 1/4 cup coconut milk
- 1 teaspoon vanilla extract
- 1 1/2 cups all-purpose flour
- 1 teaspoon baking soda
- 1/2 teaspoon salt
- 1/2 cup shredded coconut

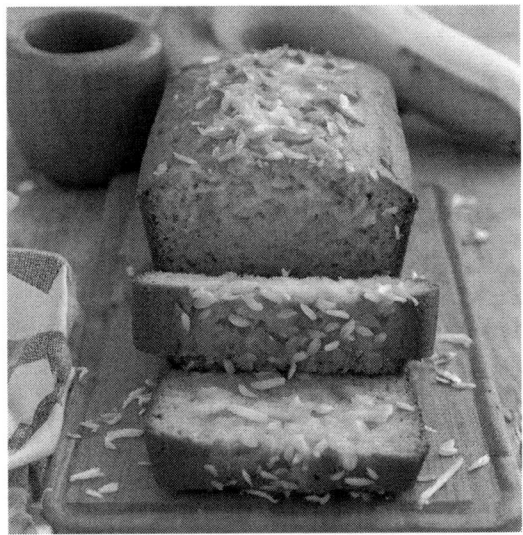

Instructions:
1. In a large bowl, combine mashed bananas, coconut oil, coconut sugar, eggs, coconut milk, and vanilla extract.
2. Stir in flour, baking soda, salt, and shredded coconut until just combined.
3. Pour the batter into a greased loaf pan that fits inside your Instant Pot.
4. Pour 1 cup of water into the Instant Pot and place the trivet inside. Set the loaf pan on the trivet.
5. Close the lid, set the valve to sealing, and cook on Manual High Pressure for 50 minutes.
6. Allow natural pressure release for 10 minutes, then quick release any remaining pressure.
7. Remove the bread and let cool before slicing.

Nutrition Info (Per Serving):
- Calories: 210
- Protein: 3g
- Fat: 10g
- Carbohydrates: 28g
- Fiber: 2g
- Serving Size: 8 servings
- Cooking Time: 60 minutes total

8-WEEK MEAL PLAN

Week 1
Day 1
- **Breakfast:** Vanilla Rice Pudding
- **Lunch:** Lemon Herb Chicken and Rice
- **Dinner:** Beef Stew with Root Vegetables

Day 2
- **Breakfast:** Apple and Walnut Breakfast Quinoa
- **Lunch:** Herbed Chicken Salad
- **Dinner:** Turmeric Coconut Basmati Rice with Parsley and Lemon Cod

Day 3
- **Breakfast:** Quinoa Apple Cinnamon Breakfast Bowl
- **Lunch:** Instant Pot Moroccan Vegetable Tagine
- **Dinner:** Ginger-Lime Cauliflower Rice with Grilled Chicken

Day 4
- **Breakfast:** Pear and Cardamom Steel-cut Oats
- **Lunch:** Zucchini Noodles with Olive Oil and Herbs
- **Dinner:** Instant Pot Lemon Pepper Cod

Day 5
- **Breakfast:** Coconut Rice Pudding
- **Lunch:** Balsamic Glazed Pork Tenderloin
- **Dinner:** Herbed Quinoa and Vegetable Stuffed Peppers

Day 6
- **Breakfast:** Lemon and Herb Quinoa Breakfast Pilaf
- **Lunch:** Instant Pot Kale and Potato Soup
- **Dinner:** Rosemary Infused Lamb Stew

Day 7
- **Breakfast:** Buckwheat Banana Pancakes
- **Lunch:** Carrot and Cumin Soup
- **Dinner:** Instant Pot Poached Pears with Maple Blondies for dessert

Week 2

Day 8
- **Breakfast:** Ginger Poached Rhubarb
- **Lunch:** Vegetable Frittata
- **Dinner:** Saffron Poached Figs

Day 9
- **Breakfast:** Pumpkin Spice Oatmeal
- **Lunch:** Lemon-Basil Shrimp Over Zoodles
- **Dinner:** Sticky Ginger Pudding

Day 10
- **Breakfast:** Mint and Lime Infused Mango
- **Lunch:** Turkey and Sweet Potato Breakfast Casserole
- **Dinner:** Instant Pot Spiced Apple Cider Chicken

Day 11
- **Breakfast:** Blueberry Millet Porridge
- **Lunch:** Savory Mushroom and Rice Breakfast Bowls
- **Dinner:** Coconut Custard

Day 12
- **Breakfast:** Spiced Peach Custard
- **Lunch:** Instant Pot Berry Compote with yogurt
- **Dinner:** Cinnamon Applesauce with Sage and Butter Turkey Breast

Day 13
- **Breakfast:** Banana Coconut Bread
- **Lunch:** Root Vegetable Medley
- **Dinner:** Instant Pot Fennel Chicken

Day 14
- **Breakfast:** Zucchini Brownies
- **Lunch:** Beef Stroganoff with Coconut Cream
- **Dinner:** Instant Pot Cabbage Rolls

Week 3

Day 15
- **Breakfast:** Instant Pot Lemon Thyme Chicken
- **Lunch:** Maple-Poached Pears
- **Dinner:** Garlic-Infused Olive Oil Drizzled Cod

Day 16
- **Breakfast:** Pumpkin Spice Cake
- **Lunch:** Parsley-Garlic Pork Chops
- **Dinner:** Peach Crumble

Day 17
- **Breakfast:** Quinoa Vegetable Pilaf
- **Lunch:** Instant Pot Moroccan Vegetable Tagine
- **Dinner:** Instant Pot Maple-Glazed Chicken

Day 18
- **Breakfast:** Saffron Vegetable Couscous
- **Lunch:** Instant Pot Tarragon Chicken
- **Dinner:** Apple and Cranberry Crisp

Day 19
- **Breakfast:** Minty Pea Soup
- **Lunch:** Herbed Quinoa and Vegetable Stuffed Peppers
- **Dinner:** Turkey Meatball Soup

Day 20
- **Breakfast:** Sticky Ginger Pudding
- **Lunch:** Bok Choy and Shiitake Mushroom Stir-Fry
- **Dinner:** Instant Pot Spiced Apple Cider Chicken

Day 21
- **Breakfast:** Vanilla Rice Pudding
- **Lunch:** Savory Mushroom and Rice Breakfast Bowls
- **Dinner:** Rosemary Infused Lamb Stew

Week 4

Day 22
- **Breakfast:** Peachy Keen Quinoa
- **Lunch:** Carrot Ginger Soup
- **Dinner:** Lemon Garlic Shrimp and Asparagus

Day 23
- **Breakfast:** Coconut Custard
- **Lunch:** Instant Pot Spaghetti Squash and Meat Sauce
- **Dinner:** Beef and Sweet Potato Stew

Day 24
- **Breakfast:** Apple and Walnut Breakfast Quinoa
- **Lunch:** Turkey and Pumpkin Chili
- **Dinner:** Savory Chicken and Rice Congee

Day 25
- **Breakfast:** Ginger-infused Millet Porridge
- **Lunch:** Zucchini and Basil Risotto
- **Dinner:** Instant Pot Poached Pears

Day 26
- **Breakfast:** Quinoa Apple Cinnamon Breakfast Bowl
- **Lunch:** Parsley and Lemon Cod
- **Dinner:** Herb-infused Breakfast Polenta

Day 27
- **Breakfast:** Pear and Cardamom Steel-cut Oats
- **Lunch:** Instant Pot Kale and Potato Soup
- **Dinner:** Maple-Poached Pears

Day 28
- **Breakfast:** Coconut Rice Pudding
- **Lunch:** Zucchini Noodles with Olive Oil and Herbs
- **Dinner:** Herb-Infused Turkey Breast

Week 5

Day 29
- **Breakfast:** Banana Coconut Bread
- **Lunch:** Lemon-Basil Shrimp Over Zoodles
- **Dinner:** Instant Pot Moroccan Vegetable Tagine

Day 30
- **Breakfast:** Minty Pea Soup
- **Lunch:** Sticky Ginger Pudding
- **Dinner:** Instant Pot Spiced Apple Cider Chicken

Day 31
- **Breakfast:** Blueberry Millet Porridge
- **Lunch:** Savory Mushroom and Rice Breakfast Bowls
- **Dinner:** Coconut Custard

Day 32
- **Breakfast:** Spiced Peach Custard
- **Lunch:** Instant Pot Berry Compote with yogurt
- **Dinner:** Cinnamon Applesauce with Sage and Butter Turkey Breast

Day 33
- **Breakfast:** Zucchini Brownies
- **Lunch:** Root Vegetable Medley
- **Dinner:** Instant Pot Fennel Chicken

Day 34
- **Breakfast:** Ginger Poached Rhubarb
- **Lunch:** Vegetable Frittata
- **Dinner:** Saffron Poached Figs

Day 35
- **Breakfast:** Pumpkin Spice Oatmeal
- **Lunch:** Turkey and Sweet Potato Breakfast Casserole
- **Dinner:** Sticky Ginger Pudding

Week 6

Day 36
- **Breakfast:** Instant Pot Lemon Thyme Chicken
- **Lunch:** Maple-Poached Pears
- **Dinner:** Garlic-Infused Olive Oil Drizzled Cod

Day 37
- **Breakfast:** Pumpkin Spice Cake
- **Lunch:** Parsley-Garlic Pork Chops
- **Dinner:** Peach Crumble

Day 38
- **Breakfast:** Quinoa Vegetable Pilaf
- **Lunch:** Instant Pot Moroccan Vegetable Tagine
- **Dinner:** Instant Pot Maple-Glazed Chicken

Day 39
- **Breakfast:** Saffron Vegetable Couscous
- **Lunch:** Instant Pot Tarragon Chicken
- **Dinner:** Apple and Cranberry Crisp

Day 40
- **Breakfast:** Minty Pea Soup
- **Lunch:** Herbed Quinoa and Vegetable Stuffed Peppers
- **Dinner:** Turkey Meatball Soup

Day 41
- **Breakfast:** Sticky Ginger Pudding
- **Lunch:** Bok Choy and Shiitake Mushroom Stir-Fry
- **Dinner:** Instant Pot Spiced Apple Cider Chicken

Day 42
- **Breakfast:** Vanilla Rice Pudding
- **Lunch:** Savory Mushroom and Rice Breakfast Bowls
- **Dinner:** Rosemary Infused Lamb Stew

Week 7

Day 43
- **Breakfast:** Pear and Ginger Jam on gluten-free toast
- **Lunch:** Beef Stroganoff with Coconut Cream
- **Dinner:** Instant Pot Lemon Pepper Cod

Day 44
- **Breakfast:** Spiced Peach Custard
- **Lunch:** Instant Pot Kale and Potato Soup
- **Dinner:** Turkey and Pumpkin Chili

Day 45
- **Breakfast:** Coconut Rice Pudding
- **Lunch:** Herbed Quinoa and Vegetable Stuffed Peppers
- **Dinner:** Instant Pot Poached Pears

Day 46
- **Breakfast:** Ginger-infused Millet Porridge
- **Lunch:** Zucchini Noodles with Olive Oil and Herbs
- **Dinner:** Herb-Infused Turkey Breast

Day 47
- **Breakfast:** Buckwheat Banana Pancakes
- **Lunch:** Instant Pot Moroccan Vegetable Tagine
- **Dinner:** Lemon Garlic Shrimp and Asparagus

Day 48
- **Breakfast:** Quinoa Apple Cinnamon Breakfast Bowl
- **Lunch:** Sticky Ginger Pudding
- **Dinner:** Balsamic Glazed Pork Tenderloin

Day 49
- **Breakfast:** Pear and Cardamom Steel-cut Oats
- **Lunch:** Vegetable Frittata
- **Dinner:** Instant Pot Spaghetti Squash and Meat Sauce

Week 8

Day 50
- **Breakfast:** Pumpkin Spice Cake
- **Lunch:** Lemon-Basil Shrimp Over Zoodles
- **Dinner:** Instant Pot Spiced Apple Cider Chicken

Day 51
- **Breakfast:** Minty Pea Soup
- **Lunch:** Savory Chicken and Rice Congee
- **Dinner:** Garlic-Infused Olive Oil Drizzled Cod

Day 52
- **Breakfast:** Blueberry Millet Porridge
- **Lunch:** Instant Pot Berry Compote with yogurt
- **Dinner:** Saffron Poached Figs

Day 53
- **Breakfast:** Spiced Peach Custard
- **Lunch:** Root Vegetable Medley
- **Dinner:** Instant Pot Fennel Chicken

Day 54
- **Breakfast:** Zucchini Brownies
- **Lunch:** Instant Pot Kale and Potato Soup
- **Dinner:** Herb-Infused Turkey Breast

Day 55
- **Breakfast:** Ginger Poached Rhubarb
- **Lunch:** Beef Stroganoff with Coconut Cream
- **Dinner:** Rosemary Infused Lamb Stew

Day 56
- **Breakfast:** Pumpkin Spice Oatmeal
- **Lunch:** Turkey and Sweet Potato Breakfast Casserole
- **Dinner:** Sticky Ginger Pudding

SCAN THE QR CODE BELOW TO GET A SURPRISE BONUS!

If you would love to have a one-on-one consultation session with Kingsley Klopp, kindly reach out to us at kloppkingsley@gmail.com

Printed in Dunstable, United Kingdom